LIVING WITH
CROHN'S &
COLITIS
COOKBOOK

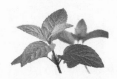

Nutritional Guidance, Meal Plans,
and Over 100 Recipes for Improved
Health and Wellness

Dede Cummings

Foreword by Sarah Choueiry

Introduction by Jessica Black, ND

))) hatherleigh

Hatherleigh Press is committed to preserving and protecting the natural resources of the earth. Environmentally responsible and sustainable practices are embraced within the company's mission statement.

Visit us at www.hatherleighpress.com and register online for free offers, discounts, special events, and more.

Living with Crohn's & Colitis Cookbook
Text copyright © 2014 Dede Cummings

Library of Congress Cataloging-in-Publication Data is available upon request.
ISBN: 978-1-57826-510-7

Cover and Interior Design by Dede Cummings

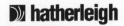

www.hatherleighpress.com

Printed in the United States
19

CONTENTS

FOREWORD

*L*iving with Crohn's and Colitis Cookbook is a great first step for anyone with inflammatory bowel disease (IBD) who would like to explore a change in their diet and nutrition to better their health. This cookbook, written by Dede Cummings, a fellow Crohn's patient, features tips on living a more holistic lifestyle by looking at the person as a whole and learning how to deal with all aspects of their condition. It is filled with practical, accessible, and up-to-date knowledge that will assist someone with IBD in exploring alternative ways to achieve their health goals.

Everyone with IBD is different; this is what makes us unique and a bit challenging. We are responsible for finding what works for each of us. We must educate, explore and implement what is given to us and make it our own. What may work for one person with IBD may not work for another.

Being a Crohnie myself, I know it can be daunting when first trying to navigate your diet and nutrition, which is why I support this book and was honored to contribute to it. One of the first books that helped me find alternative methods to treat my Crohn's was written by Dede. That book, *Living with Crohn's & Colitis: A Comprehensive Naturopathic Guide for Complete Digestive Wellness,* co-authored by Dede's naturopath, Jessica Black, ND, opened my eyes to a world I did not know existed.

I understand how overwhelming it may seem when first diagnosed with Crohn's disease or ulcerative colitis. I know this from my own experiences as well as from the many stories I have heard through my foundation, The Crohn's Journey Foundation. Every day

I hear at least one new story of someone taken aback and confused by a diagnosis they had never heard of before. When I was first diagnosed with Crohn's disease, I did not take it seriously. It was not until September 2012, when I was hospitalized and felt like I could not survive another day, that I really accepted that this was a serious disease. I wanted guidance on how to help myself get better and realized in order to do this, I had to look beyond western medicine. Looking back at that time, armed with the knowledge I now have, I see the necessity of a whole mind, body approach..

After reaching out to Dede, I continued my research and began to reach out to other holistic and alternative practitioners and advocates. I pursued my foundation and made it a mission to teach others who were also struggling with Crohn's and IBD that there are other options besides medication—it is a whole soul, body, and mind approach. I wanted to emphasize that yes, *diet* does matter.

I am very passionate about holistic approaches to IBD, and that is why I feel this book is needed. Remember; take what you find in here as an outline to achieving your health goals. This book should be a road map where you fill in the blanks and figure out what works for you and what doesn't. I hope this will inspire you, as it has me.

Sending love to all your bellies,
SARAH CHOUEIRY
Founder, The Crohn's Journey Foundation

INTRODUCTION

To LEAD A HEALTHY LIFESTYLE, we must consider our relationship with food to be a vital part of survival. If we exist because of the nutrients we consume, our health is reflected by what we eat on a daily basis. There are many important aspects to consider when fueling the body. In current society, our understanding of food for survival and health has declined over generations. Processing and handling has changed our relationship with food and has even altered our taste for food. We have become accustomed to the buttery, rich, sweet flavors of processed foods and the more we eat these types of foods, the more we crave them. Our hunger becomes insatiable when we eat processed, unnatural foods. Obesity and weight gain plague our population, thus contributing to many chronic illnesses. If only the way we ate gave our bodies a better sense of satiety, we could feed our bodies without overeating.

Many generations prior, individuals had to hunt and gather to obtain food. In addition, the food they ate was of utmost freshness and was extremely nutrient-dense, without the added calories, sugar, and fat contained in the foods we eat today.

Earlier generations also experienced stress very differently from the stress we face today. Years ago, stressors were consistently related to survival and were often met with physical demands. In this sense, stress was important because it provided individuals the chemicals needed to move to a safer location or run after their hunt. Due to our present-day sedentary habits and because stress is consistently related to symptoms and flare-ups of digestive disorders, finding

3

ways to reduce stress is essential to digestion and long-term wellness for all sufferers.

Earlier in history, when we had to hunt or grow our own food, we appreciated its worth and its gift to us as life-giving power. We were mindful as we shared this food together with our families. It is my assumption that if we once again had to roam, hunt, and gather to obtain food, our culture would be much more appreciative of the food we consume and we would take the time to appreciate the eating process. We can learn something important from indigenous cultures; to honor and cherish the earth for producing our food and allowing us to be nourished. A simple prayer or reflection before meals can change the intent during a family meal. Concentrate on keeping calm, chew your food slowly, and pay attention to the food you are eating. Taking the time to do this during family meals can change how you digest.

It is presumptuous to assume that we can return to those times of hunting and gathering. However, as a society, we can make large efforts to pay more attention to our eating and lifestyle habits. Lifestyle habits can make the difference between disease and wellness. From food choices, exercise, and meal-time habits to meditation and giving thanks, we can make differences in our health, no matter what plagues us.

Serendipity—when two people meet on the street and know they were meant to be there at that precise time in order to meet each other. To know that coming together for them meant something so much more than the sideward glance they shared before enlightenment. In many ways, I feel that my meeting Dede Cummings has been serendipitous.

In working with Dede Cummings, I have learned about the grace and beauty she encompasses in her approach to health and wellness. What Dede suggests in *Living with Crohn's & Colitis Cookbook* is about simplifying foods and engaging in more meditative habits; practices that our society as a whole has nearly forgotten. My history with Dede suggests a kind of sweet serendipity that catapulted us forward into co-authoring a book together. Our energetic "meeting" really started when Dede's doctor gave her a copy of my book, *The Anti-Inflammation Diet and Recipe Book*. After using it and enjoying it, Dede contacted me and asked if we could write a book together. We decided to work on it, but due to our busy schedules, the idea was slowly pushed to the back of my mind as I carried on through my daily life. Then a few years later, Dede announced she had everything ready to go for us to begin writing and we began the incredible journey of working on our first book together, *Living with Crohn's and Colitis* (I say "first book" because I envision us working in tandem for years to come).

Through the process of transferring the manuscript back and forth over thousands of emails, we found that our views on health, meditation, lifestyle, and diet paralleled each other's without challenge, even though we had never met. So, actually our serendipitous meeting was at a book signing after we had already finished our manuscript together!

In the *Living with Crohn's & Colitis Cookbook*, Dede does a wonderful job of simply bringing us through IBD and other digestive disorders, and improving our understanding of the medical thought process behind diagnosis. Interestingly, Dede was wrongly diagnosed initially, which often happens when someone suffers from gastrointestinal problems without a discoverable cause. Dede has a very accessible and personal writing style that brings you into a more positive state of mind. You may find yourself thinking, "I can do that," or "I really am going to feel better." This is a powerful part of healing. A person cannot heal if he or she doesn't believe it. Among my patients, those most likely to have the quickest recovery tend to have the best attitude, a good sense of humor, a balanced lifestyle, and an affinity for exercising.

It is extremely important to consider that our relationship with food will affect how we heal. Food is central to the entire chasm of living beings. Practically, food provides nutrients for our body's fuel. It is more central than you may realize. Food stimulates conversations and initiates friendships and relationships. Food is everywhere. Think of how often you may have scheduled a social activity that involved food in one way or another. Dates, having people over, parties, ceremonies, going out after work, going to a friend's house for dinner, lunch meetings, breakfast meetings—these are just a few examples of the many ways that we interact with each other around food.

So why is it that societal food choices are not typically healthy and nourishing? We have veered far from our roots in our food choices and farming practices. Research has shown that poor food choices affect health outcomes for the future. There is a direct correlation between fats, sugars, and processed foods and illness. There is also a direct relationship between healthy foods such as vegetables, fruits, nuts, seeds, and other high-fiber foods and a decrease in negative health outcomes. It is being proven in the research, now we just need to start listening and making changes in our own lives.

As hard as change is, it can be liberating and exhilarating. Increasing healthy foods in your diet is a good start, and Dede has done a great job of presenting us with delicious recipes in a way that enables us to still savor food, without having to sacrifice taste.

I am positive that you will be thanking yourself for picking up this book and will enjoy putting into practice some of the suggestions that Dede offers in the following pages.

Jessica Black, N.D.
Author of *The Anti-Inflammation Diet and Recipe Book* and co-author of *Living with Crohn's and Colitis: A Comprehensive Naturopathic Guide for Complete Digestive Wellness*

AUTHOR'S NOTE

I WAS 45 when I learned about the disease that was going to change my life. Up until then, my life had been largely without significant personal struggle. As an adult, I had celebrated the birth of three healthy babies and enjoyed a career that I loved, working in the world of book publishing. Some travel, fluency in another language, a college degree, and an outwardly happy family formed the nucleus around a marriage to my college boyfriend. Under the surface were family tensions and the death of one of my closest friends, a doctor, from breast cancer at the age of 41, which left me confused and somewhat prone to depression. As is evident in my story, however, I masked the pain of emotional distress and physical trauma quite well: I was a high-functioning professional woman with a career in book publishing as a designer.

After my diagnosis with Crohn's disease, I did not set out to actually write a book; instead I was keeping a food journal, which is really important for sufferers of IBD, both young and old. For an entire week, my naturopathic doctor suggested writing in a journal all the symptoms my body had and everything I was doing and eating during that time. I was told to be sure to record all symptoms, from the most minor crick in the neck to low back pain, to headaches, to diarrhea. By doing this, I began to learn how my body was trying to communicate to me: I began to listen to my body more and more, and then it became easier for me to notice these connections.

In 2006, after coming home from my bowel resection, my food journal began more as "notes to my surgeon," that became somewhat

7

humorous and sarcastic (for example, "Well, Dr. H, you told me to keep a food journal so here goes . . . this is going to be really boring since I now eat practically the same thing every day!").

Later on, as my food journal progressed, I began to explore how and why I started to have symptoms and how having Crohn's disease, with some ulcerative colitis as well, was affecting my life, and the so-called "journal" took on a life of its own.

My publishing story is not unique: I wanted to buy a book that would help me as a lifestyle guide for the inflammatory bowel disease (IBD) I suffered from. I searched for a book that would incorporate both the knowledge that comes from Western medicine (i.e., high-tech, science based), along with a naturopathic approach that could readily be integrated into a healthy, active life.

This kind of book didn't exist in 2006, so I set out to write my first book, *Living with Crohn's & Colitis: A Comprehensive Naturo-pathic Guide for Complete Digestive Wellness*. What sets my first book apart, I think, is that it explains the disease, and attempts to help sufferers live with the disease, both by understanding it better and also, more practically, by providing lifestyle strategies (such as yoga, recipes, etc.).

By the spring of 2010, *Living with Crohn's & Colitis* was released and began to stimulate very positive reactions. A writer for *Prevention* magazine's story "4 Screening Tests Women Fear" interviewed me and the article was reprinted widely; another article about my struggle to overcome Crohn's disease appeared in MORE magazine, and my co-author Dr. Jessica Black, and I have since been on numerous radio shows. I built a website, started a blog, and began Twitter and Facebook pages, which have increased exposure, and book sales are growing with the book now helping many patients, medical professionals, and caregivers alike.

Ultimately, for me, although the book that emerged is mainly about disease and recovery, it is also about confronting pain courageously and living life to celebrate it.

This book is my story, but it is also a way for me to aid others who are either newly diagnosed with these lonely and debilitating diseases of the bowel or who have a loved one who is living with inflammatory bowel disease. The book is also a wellness guide and I am grateful to my co-author, Dr. Jessica Black, who offered the perfect balance to my patient story by offering a comprehensive naturopathic approach to achieving and maintaining health and longevity.

In the spirit of hope, espoused by Jerome Groopman, M.D., in his groundbreaking book, *Anatomy of Hope: How People Prevail in the Face of Illness* I offer this companion cookbook to our readers, as a way to lend more support and compassion, and yes, hope. It is hope, I also believe, that a patient truly needs in order to survive and even to thrive.

I hope this cookbook becomes a vital and inspirational addition to everyone's kitchen bookshelf!

Dede Cummings
May 5, 2014
West Brattleboro, Vermont

CHAPTER 1

Learning to Love
and Heal Your Body

IN MY FIRST BOOK, *Living with Crohn's & Colitis: A Compre-*
hensive Naturopathic Guide for Complete Digestive Wellness, Dr.
Jessica Black and I argue that eating well is key in prevention and
treatment of digestive diseases, including Crohn's disease, ulcerative
colitis, and other diseases of the gut. Why are autoimmune diseases
on the rise across the board in the world today? Some theories
include the advent of refrigeration and the overuse of antibiotics.
However the basic fact that our bodies have trouble digesting
over-refined foods is argument for a simple diet that is easy to cook,
to chew, and to digest: for example, steamed or roasted veggies, rice,
and some protein (tofu or chicken). Our first book advocated an
anti-inflammation diet, joining a farmshare/CSA, slowing down,
and de-stressing life. Now, with *Living with Crohn's & Colitis Cook-*
book, we will guide you step-by-step in integrating this simple and
nutritious diet into your everyday life.

IBD ON THE RISE

Why are people suffering from the debilitating effects of Inflammatory Bowel Disease (IBD) across the board in the United States, and
in other developed countries?

It is no secret that ulcerative colitis and Crohn's disease are on the rise, and a new study traces how a typical Western diet that is high in saturated fats (found in dairy products, baked goods, and processed foods) may increase the chance of an imbalance in the gut microbes. According to a recent article in Scientific American's Health Blog by Katherine Harmon, Crohn's and colitis (inflammation of the large intestine that can cause pain and diarrhea) seems to run in families, but not everyone with the genetic risk gets the disease. Because of this, scientists have presumed that an environmental trigger initiates the disease.

According to Eugene Chang, a professor of medicine at the University of Chicago and co-author of a new study published in *Nature*, "Moving from elevated risk to the development of the disease seems to require a second event, which may be encountered because of our changing lifestyle."

Chang and his colleagues traced how saturated fats, particularly those from dairy, which are also present in many baked goods and processed foods, can change the composition of naturally harmless bacteria in the gut. As the balance of bacteria species shifts, it can trigger an immune response that results in inflammation and tissue damage.

The word "inflammatory" literally means relating to or causing inflammation of a part of the body. In Dr. Chang's study, comparisons were studied between a group of mice with a genetic predisposition for intestinal disease which were fed a diet high in dairy and saturated fats, versus a group with the same genetic predisposition which were fed a diet low in saturated fats.

The mice that were genetically predisposed and fed a diet high in dairy and saturated fat developed a harmful bacteria (with an extremely poetic name), *Bilophila wadsworthia,* which is also found in patients with intestinal diseases. In fact, the team at the University of Chicago found that the mice with the increase in harmful bacteria went on to develop an immuno-activated response that created subsequent inflammation.

What can we learn from this study? First of all, I want to applaud Dr. Chang and his team, as well as the excellent reporting by Katherine Harmon and the publishers of *Nature* and *Scientific American.* Those of us who live *daily* with inflammatory bowel disease are anticipating that this knowledge will help us find a cure that doesn't depend on drugs to suppress the entire immune system (a treatment that often creates other health problems).

WHAT CAN WE DO NOW?

As a layperson and author who struggles with Crohn's-Colitis, I follow blogs and scientific journals with the zeal of a medical student doing a GI rotation. Call me crazy, but I am *not* going to sit around getting sicker and waiting for the doctors to complete long term trials and simulations. We can start by eating a simple, structured diet; what I like to refer to as a diet where we "eat food with one ingredient."

Next, we can keep a food journal. Start by eliminating dairy for three days and see if that helps, then record what you eat—usually small frequent meals are best: oatmeal in the morning, followed by a hard-boiled egg at 10:30, lunch is a spinach salad with turkey and a rice cake, afternoon snack can be raisins and almonds or carrots and pure hummus with garlic and lemon, and dinner is beans and rice or baked chicken or fish with steamed broccoli. (All of these are just suggestions, if tolerated, as everyone is different!)

I have not eaten wheat for seven years, which has been of great benefit. Though I still love dairy products, like cheese and yogurt, I gave them up a year ago. I recommend cutting back on dairy, switching to lower fat cheeses like provolone, and making your own yogurt by following the Specific Carbohydrate Diet (SCD) book, *Breaking the Vicious Cycle* by Elaine Gottschall.

Adding probiotics to your diet with a daily supplement is also a great way to help balance the gut microbial balance. I use All-Flora Probiotics by Metangenics. When I am traveling, I use the great

Jarrow product, Jarro-Dophilus EPS, which has 5 billion organisms per capsule.

Don't forget to exercise, eat a balanced diet with small frequent meals, keep a food journal daily, get lots of sleep (eight hours is recommended), and add holistic and complementary treatments to your lifestyle, such as acupuncture, daily yoga, and meditation, as outlined in my previous book *Living with Crohn's & Colitis*.

DEDE'S BACKSTORY

I love to travel and left home when I was eighteen to live in Europe by myself for a year. I settled in Vienna, Austria, and loved the culture and the people. The diet, however, was not the healthiest, and I gained twenty-five pounds by subsisting on Würst, bread, and of course, beer. I remember, when I came back from Europe, my father looked at me and said, "you've gained twice the Freshman 15, and you didn't even go to college!"

Well, here I am, many years later—with college, marriage, and three wonderful children behind me—and I have to say that the one good thing that having Crohn's disease has done is that I no longer worry about my weight, and I just eat what I can and make no apologies to anyone. My weight has stayed at around 140, which my gastroenterologist says is perfect because I eat healthy food all the time—hardly any sugar, no fried food, no wheat, and very low-fat dairy—and I exercise daily, and maintain a low-stress lifestyle.

The reason I was motivated to write this cookbook was not to talk about our American culture's unhealthy obsession with being thin as a sign of success; I wrote it to talk about the opposite—I hope the recipes in this book will encourage you to learn to eat, cook (and even grow!) healthy food, love your body and cherish your family, and take responsibility for your own health and education.

I say this because for years, I wallowed in self-pitying behavior during my Crohn's flares, which occurred monthly and had the nasty habit of coinciding with my menstrual period. I used to crawl into bed and sometimes cry quietly, so as not to disturb my kids. After driving the kids to school (during one of these flares), I would frequently pull over to the side of the road in my car, and just put my head on the steering wheel and sob. It took me years to ask for help, and by the time I was finally diagnosed, my disease had basically devoured my terminal ileum, for it was beyond repair due to repeated flares leading to scarring.

So having first had symptoms of ulcerative colitis (I have this, too!) after I returned from Vienna (remember my unhealthy lifestyle, horrible diet, and self-loathing attitude?), fast forward to 2006, to when I was admitted to the ER with a stomach the size of a basketball and a severely impacted bowel that was about to rupture. I finally admitted that I was one sick person and I needed help.

That was my first step toward getting well. In the past, I would constantly think about what I could or could not eat to stay thin and be attractive. I smoked cigarettes to curb my appetite and utilized the diuretic aid that nicotine provides; I also worked all the time and exercised in fits and starts, and tried to diet, off and on, but always gained the weight back.

Having my kids and going through childbirth helped me let go of inhibitions and was a great release for me. I always wanted to be trim and fit and "in control." One thing I've learned from having Crohn's is that sometimes when you lie on the cold and smelly bathroom floor with your arms wrapped around the toilet crying and in pain, you are clearly *not* in control!

LEARNING TO LOVE AND HEAL YOUR BODY

After Jessica Black, N.D. and I came out with our *Living with Crohn's and Colitis* book, I was interviewed by Linda Sparrowe, a writer from *Yoga International,* who wrote:

"A disordered body image isn't always about weight, of course. Dede Cummings, a graphic designer from Vermont, remembers the time she was in a yoga class practicing handstand and her shirt came up, revealing a huge scar on her belly that she hated and felt ashamed of—a result of multiple surgeries. Her yoga teacher told her she was beautiful. 'But my scar,' she said. 'Your scar is beautiful, too,' he said. 'It's a part of who you are.'"

So for my fellow Crohn's disease and ulcerative colitis readers, and people who love you who may also be reading, I urge you to *let go*, and by that I mean ask for help, but also study everything you can about your disease and admit you have a serious disease that can even lead to death. Don't be polite at potluck dinner parties; at restaurants, ask for gluten-free pasta or rice, well-steamed fresh local veggies (especially available in summer), and baked fish specifically made for you if the menu doesn't have easy-to-digest food you know you can tolerate. Don't be afraid to take control of your health and get your life back on track—it *is* possible to enjoy an active fulfilling, healthy life with IBD!

HOW THIS BOOK CAN HELP

In this book, I do not offer strict diet rules for "this or that digestive disease." Instead, I offer up my own tried-and-true nutritional suggestions based on my interpretation of current medical research (remember, I follow gastroenterology papers, studies, and the like, with the zeal of a pre-medical student!), and personal stories that will, hopefully, help people cope, learn about their disease, and thrive!

The specific types of information you can expect to find in the following pages include tips for food shopping, a guide to keeping a food journal, and recipes for when you have a flare, plus recipes for typical daily life. I wrote this book to complement the work Jessica Black, N.D., and I presented in our first book, and I hope that you will be able to read that first or concurrently with this cookbook.

As you read, you will find recipes for making basic meals that are not complex and that use simple ingredients, plus staples that include how to make your own home-cooked chicken soup, rice, beans, guacamole, almond milk, and more.

I have also included some basic tips for food shopping along with information about how to avoid pesticide-tainted fruits and vegetables, joining a farmshare (CSA), and creating your own vegetable garden.

One of my basic premises in this cookbook is to help you plan and create an individualized diet just for you or for someone you love or care for who has inflammatory bowel disease. A daily food journal forms the foundation of the plan as do other holistic lifestyle activities including getting daily exercise and enough sleep, practicing yoga and meditation to calm your brain and relieve stress, and other health-promoting techniques you will learn about.

The recipes in this book are really unique and have been approved by many of my "Crohnie" and "UC-er" friends! There is a very strong community of IBD/IBS people out there (I honestly don't like to use the word "sufferers" due to the negativity of the word), who share recipes, and I list many websites and places where you can get support.

It is my hope that those with Crohn's or colitis, and variations of these diseases, and even those diagnosed with Irritable Bowel Syndrome (IBS), will be able to benefit from taking control of their own diet through using this cookbook.

CHAPTER 2

Creating Balance in Your Diet

WHAT ARE Crohn's disease and ulcerative colitis? These diseases are part of a category of illnesses known as inflammatory bowel disease (IBD). Inflammatory bowel disease (IBD) is the general name for diseases that cause swelling in the intestines. A regulatory border within the body uses chemical messengers and hormones as keys to allow access to important chemicals and deny access to unwanted materials. The gastrointestinal tract is one of the most important regulatory borders we have in the body. It functions to allow healthful nutrients or beneficial bacteria in and to keep out unwanted microorganisms or larger food particles that may harm or overload the system. Inflammatory bowel disease (IBD) stems from a confusion, or misunderstanding, of the mucosal immune system function in the intestine. When this confusion occurs, the intestinal lining can begin mounting reactions against normally harmless bacteria, foods, and so on, and inflammation occurs in the colon as a result.

The causes of inflammation for those with Crohn's, ulcerative colitis (UC), and other forms of IBD are complex, involving a number of factors. These include one's environment, microbial balance, genetics, stress and emotional health, diet and lifestyle habits, and immunological factors.

Although the cause of IBD is not clear, one can learn what causes inflammation for each individual and then use this knowledge to improve lifestyle habits and create balance in their diet and in their life.

GUT MICROBES MAY PLAY A ROLE IN CROHN'S DISEASE

Did you know that there is more bacteria in the gut than there are human cells in the body? According to a recent NPR article, research involving more than 1,500 patients found that people with Crohn's disease had a less diverse populations of gut microbes. Taking probiotics is a good way to help balance the gut microflora. There are over 100 trillion microoganisms and hundreds of different species in the human bowel. The bacteria in the gut helps keep pathogens from causing harm. Studies are currently being done, and the results are not consistent, but even Harvard Medical School has asserted that "probiotic therapy may also help people with Crohn's disease and irritable bowel syndrome."

Ramnik Xavier, M.D., Ph.D., of Massachusetts General Hospital in Boston, who led the research, which was published in the journal *Cell, Host & Microbe*, stated that in addition to having less diversity in their gut microbes, the Crohn's patients had fewer bacteria that have been associated with reduced inflammation and more bacteria associated with increased inflammation. "There's the possibility that we might be able to identify [some] sort of super-probiotics that might be able to correct the gut back to the healthy state," Xavier says.

The term, "probiotics," comes from *pro* and *biota*, meaning "for life." The new term and products called "super probiotics" that have recently come on the market is certainly worth watching and the next steps taken by medical research may reveal them to aid in a variety of illnesses. For centuries, cultures have eaten fermented foods, such as yogurt, which transfers live bacteria into the gut. Here in America, we have lagged behind other countries, perhaps because the idea of ingesting "bacteria" is anathema to our culture's fixation on antibiotic "cleanliness."

This fixation on taking a pill, or antibiotic, is currently changing drastically with the Centers for Disease Control (CDC) instructing doctors to wait before routinely prescribing antibiotics. As far as rushing out to spend extra money on super probiotics, it is advisable to wait and follow Dr. Xavier and others in their research. Ingesting natural probiotics (commonly called "pre-biotics" if they are ingested as food products) is not harmful at all and may in fact be beneficial as studies now show, especially for infants and women with vaginal infections.

According to Harvard Medical School, "The best case for probiotic therapy has been in the treatment of diarrhea. Controlled trials have shown that *Lactobacillus rhamnosus GG* can shorten the course of infectious diarrhea in infants and children." Ingesting probiotics and taking a supplement if you have inflammatory bowel disease seems like a prudent approach to aid in healing the gut.

Although there is no dietary "cure" for IBD, eating well can make a major difference for those living with the symptoms. Choosing the right foods and avoiding the wrong ones can help reduce (and possibly eliminate) the occurrence of symptoms and lead to a more normally functioning digestive tract.

By shifting to an IBD-friendly diet, the body will not only be receiving rich nutrients, but will also become more regulated, allowing the digestive tract muscles to relax and easily break down the food.

Increasing your intake of the right fruits, vegetables, grains, and meats while staying away from fatty, sugary, and stomach-straining foods, can lead to better well-being with less symptoms and more time to just be you; and, hopefully, keep your health on track for years to come.

The dietary suggestions outlined in these introductory chapters will show you how to create a meal plan that will steer clear of "trigger" foods, which can be a setback on your quest for a healthy and symptom-free diet. Keep in mind that each individual is different and not everyone will have the same reactions to certain foods. However, some people will prefer to eliminate all foods that characteristically worsen symptoms.

Speak to your GI doctor, or specialist, about the dietary guidelines below and seek his or her guidance based on your own unique symptoms and needs before beginning any dietary regimen.

If you haven't already, omit from your daily diet any foods that irritate or increase your symptoms; this can drastically improve your digestive health and regularity.

These dietary changes can be your first step towards better health:

AVOID dairy products like milk, cheese, and yogurt. Even if you're normally tolerant to these foods, the high fat content can lead to diarrhea and can increase digestive discomfort.

AVOID certain vegetables like broccoli, Brussels sprouts, cabbage, and cauliflower, which increase gas.

Note that excessive intake of fiber can also lead to gas and cramping. However, depending on your symptoms, a gradual increase of soluble fibers (such as apples, oats, and citrus fruits) and insoluble fibers (found in whole grains, bran, and most vegetables) can help relieve constipation by moving material through the digestive system. Adding a bit of ground flaxseed to your diet allows some

NOW WHAT DO YOU EAT?

Call me crazy, but I love this question! Your diet no longer includes wheat and has very little red meat, and limited dairy. You may be asking yourself, *now what do I eat?*

Make Fruits and Veggies your main course. The first step is to increase your intake of fruits and vegetables. A great way to have easy access to fresh produce is to start your own garden—my little 3 x 10 foot raised beds are producing like crazy now. (See the section at the end of this book, on page 182 for tips on creating a garden.)

Replace Wheat with Spelt or Gluten-Free Grains. People always ask me why I cannot eat wheat and I don't have a clear answer. I remember my naturopath asking me to give up wheat when I was really having digestive issues—mostly constipation and blockages—and I was horrified. "I love pizza and bagels the most," I pleaded with her. She demurred and suggested I give up wheat for three days to see if that helped my frequent bouts of arthritis due to the long-term flares of Crohn's disease that had ravaged my joints.

After three days, I was ecstatic—I had more energy, and I felt better all over, especially in my elbows and knees which were frequently arthritic. I switched to the ancient wheat grain, spelt, for my occasional wheat-fixes (though I typically use rice flour for pastas and pizza crusts). Spelt looks very similar to wheat (just ask my twenty-one-year-old son who often samples my spelt concoctions, like pizza dough and scones, and doesn't notice any difference from the same made with wheat!)

Spelt actually contains more protein than wheat, and since I limit my intake of red meat, I do like getting extra protein in my diet. In addition, the protein is easier to digest, though there is actually more gluten in spelt, which makes it an unsuitable grain for those with celiac disease. There are some wonderful gluten-free alternatives (check out "Against the Grain," a Vermont company that makes pizza and bagels!).

As far as oats are concerned, I have found this grain to be easier to digest than most other whole grains. (*Note*: I only use pure oats, not commercial oats, which are often processed with wheat. If you have celiac disease you *must* stay away from any wheat contamination.)

Eat Six Small Meals a Day. A healthy breakfast should energize you, satisfy your hunger and provide beneficial nutrients—carbohydrates, protein, vitamins, minerals, and a small amount of fat. A bowl of high quality oatmeal that has some dietary fiber with pure almond milk (see the recipe on page 77), cut-up fruit, and even a few nuts provides a lot more nutrients than an empty calorie food like that sweet roll or doughnut. In addition to lowering blood cholesterol, oatmeal can help control blood sugar and insulin sensitivity. Whole grains including oatmeal are digested more slowly than refined grains. This slower digestion leads to a gradual, steady supply of blood sugar which can keep hunger in check.

After a morning breakfast of either oatmeal or cut-up fruit and nuts with almond milk, you can plan a mid-morning snack of a boiled egg, followed by a healthy salad or soup for lunch, then a mid-afternoon snack of almond butter and carrots, followed by a vegetable-focused dinner with a side of protein.

Be Choosy with Nutrition Labels. When making diet and lifestyle choices, I always read labels carefully—sometimes the fewer ingredients on the label, the happier I am and more apt to purchase!

SOAKING NUTS

According to Foodmatters[R], soaking nuts, grains, seeds, and legumes in warm water for seven hours is a good way to get the nutritional benefits out the foods while also making them easier to digest.

Why soak nuts, grains, and seeds?
- To remove or reduce phytic acid.
- To remove or reduce tannins.

- To neutralize the enzyme inhibitors.
- To encourage the production of beneficial enzymes.
- To increase the amounts of vitamins, especially B vitamins.
- To break down gluten and make digestion easier.
- To make the proteins more readily available for absorption.
- To prevent mineral deficiencies and bone loss.
- To help neutralize toxins in the colon and keep the colon clean.
- To prevent many health diseases and conditions.

Many of us with Crohn's disease have trouble with the absorption of B vitamins and other essential minerals since our terminal ileums (the smallest end of the small intestine where it meets the large colon) are either compromised due to inflammation or scarring, or (as in my case) removed entirely. It is important to keep an eye on what food we ingest and how we ingest it to achieve maximum benefits.

WHAT CAUSES A FLARE-UP?

The short answer to what causes a flare up, is that doctors don't really know what causes IBD to begin with, and intermittent flares during the disease progression can sometimes come on without warning. Sometimes the muscles of the large colon don't contract or expand properly to aid in the digestion of food; or, rather than a mechanical problem, the patient has trouble breaking down food due to an overly sensitive gut that is prone to cause gas and bloating, or what is referred to as "Leaky Gut Syndrome" (see The Specific Carbohydrate Diet Lifestyle on page 177 in the Resources).

Current medical research looks at the beneficial biological effects of sleep and exercise on symptoms and well-being in the field of IBD. As many of us are aware, stress has a significant and impressionable influence on all diseases. In fact, stress and the hormones that are secreted in times of excess stress directly affect our health. In today's world, our lifestyles play a huge role in the prevalence of particular diseases, including IBD.

During the summer of 2013, I was freaking out because I thought I had Lyme disease, but it turns out it was a Crohn's flare-up. (Yes, I have been so happy to be in clinical remission for the past six and a half years, I'd forgotten what it was like to have a flare up!)

I originally thought I had Lyme disease because I was having stiffness and flu-like symptoms. Earlier that summer, I had a systemic flare of poison ivy and my dermatologist thinks the acute contact dermatitis actually caused my body to get out of balance, resulting in a flare-up.

DIET CHANGES FOR FLARE-UPS

Jessica K. Black, N.D., author of *The Anti-Inflammation Diet and Recipe Book*, suggests that food is a healthier way to control inflammation and reduce chronic disease than taking medications. Drugs used to reduce inflammation are either steroids or nonsteroidal anti-inflammatory drugs (NSAIDS). Taking steroids can damage the immune system and both categories of drugs can have damaging side effects. Instead, Black recommends eating anti-inflammatory foods that boost health while reducing chronic illness.

Dr. Black tells us that an important step in implementing a

personal anti-inflammatory diet is eliminating food allergens. When the dieter eats a food allergen, his or her body may stimulate the production of antibodies that can cause an inflammatory response. My basic diet now excludes caffeine, dairy, processed foods, alcohol, and trans fats. Instead I eat Specific Carbohydrate Diet (SCD) certified foods such as fresh-steamed veggies, cold water fish, and other foods that do not trigger inflammation in the gut.

Dr. Black recommends eliminating all potential allergy triggers, including:

- Caffeinated beverages
- Fried foods
- Processed foods
- Peanut butter
- Carbonated soda
- Citrus
- Wheat
- Pork
- Tomatoes

- Potatoes
- Dairy
- Sugar
- Eggs
- Shellfish
- Peanuts
- Anything that contains hydrogenated oil

After four weeks, reintroduce the eliminated items, one per week, and if no allergic symptoms occur, add the item back into your diet but note any changes in your food journal (see Chapter 4).

THE SPECIFIC CARBOHYDRATE DIET

Another great approach to education and eating is by following the Specific Carbohydrate Diet (SCD), which is a diet that helped me so much six years ago. (See Resources page 177).

With the SCD, you eliminate complex carbohydrates, lactose, sucrose, and other man-made ingredients from the digestive process, which allows the body to finally start healing. As gut flora levels start to stabilize, the reduction of irritants from undigested foods, toxins, and other man-made ingredients allows inflammation levels to retreat.

The Specific Carbohydrate Diet (SCD) is a group of foods which are grain-free, sugar-free, starch-free, and unprocessed. While removing many foods that are toxic and digestively harmful, the diet remains natural, extremely nourishing, and representative of what our ancestors ate.

Eating SCD is a way to "re-boot" your digestion and give you an overall health boost. The diet will probably have you feeling better than ever, even if you don't have any intestinal damage. But if you do need a bit of digestive support, this diet was created especially for you. Learn more about this diet at www.SCDLifestyle.com.

noodles and tortillas (note: corn is not as easily tolerated as rice flour for many with IBD).

Between flares, eat a wide variety of foods as tolerated. This includes fruits, vegetables, whole grains, lean protein, and low-fat and nonfat dairy products.

Increase your calorie and protein intake following a flare. Abdominal pain, diarrhea, and decreased appetite may have caused poor food intake. Steroids used to treat flares also can increase protein needs.

Suggestions for first foods after a flare include:

- Homemade bone broth, gradually adding chicken soup (see SCD recipe—Grandma's Chicken Soup—on page 86)
- Diluted juices (no sugar added): use 1 part juice to 3 parts water
- Banana
- Applesauce
- Canned fruit
- Oatmeal
- Plain chicken, turkey, or fish
- Cooked eggs or egg substitutes (as tolerated)
- Mashed potatoes or well-cooked rice
- Bread: It's recommended not to eat bread and grains at all (except grains made from almonds or coconut), but sometimes a slice of toast with some honey is the perfect complement to a post-flare or during-flare menu

WHAT CAN WE DO GOING FORWARD?

Additional lifestyle changes you can make to create more balance in your life can be added on after the dietary changes are implemented. Remember, everyone has different levels of tolerance for certain foods. My tolerance for cornmeal may not be the same for you, so keeping a food journal (see chapter 4) will create a good record of what you eat, when you ate it, and what the outcome was.

Grow your own food, and commute to work via bicycle or walk. We must adapt environmentally, as well as health-wise, as inflammation is the by-product of idiopathic (meaning no known cause or cure) diseases like Crohn's, colitis, and IBS. Growing your own food in organically prepared soil is not only a healthy alternative that will ultimately save you money, but also will allow you to gain confidence and enjoy the freshest vegetables possible. Riding your bicycle will not only cut down on climate-changing fossil fuel emissions (clearly a proven scientific and man-made problem globally), but it will also allow you to benefit from the added exercise.

Keep a Food Journal. Achieving balance in the gut flora and fauna is made easier when you are armed with a food journal and a list of trigger foods to avoid. You can begin to take steps to move toward a dietary basis that will encourage healthy eating for you and your whole family.

Be Patient. Many of us are on a tight budget and need to shop and save money at the same time, so it can take awhile to implement dietary changes. The way to achieve balance in one's diet doesn't happen overnight. We need to be patient when we take these first steps, and ask our GI clinics and specialists to refer us to a dietician who is really up on the latest healthy trends.

Stay Informed. What is really important is becoming educated about IBD and listening to your body. The term homeostasis, or achieving a balance in the gut microbial balance, should not be talked of only in biochemistry labs, but also in our own kitchens and small gardens, with regard to the food we purchase, grow, cook, and eat.

In the next chapter, you will find even more tips for a holistic approach to reducing IBD symptoms.

CHAPTER 3

Following a Holistic Lifestyle

N OW THAT WE ARE on our way toward better health through diet, avoiding all processed foods, and starting to feel better after only a few days, it is time to gradually introduce a more holistic lifestyle. Don't let the term "holistic lifestyle" intimidate you or deter you from your goal. A holistic lifestyle simply means to follow a multi-pronged approach to integrating healing and balance into your life, and this chapter will detail a few easy way to do this.

The main thing to remember is that it takes time to change habits, and sometimes having a tough diagnosis—like Crohn's, IBD, colitis, celiac disease, diverticular disease, and the like—can really scare us and throw us for a loop. In this chapter, I have outlined some broad-based approaches to aid in adapting a more holistic lifestyle.

TAKE CONTROL OF YOUR LIFE

Taking control of your life and learning everything you can about your autoimmune disease are good first steps. Ask questions of your doctors during interviews, and seek out local health practitioners that are recommended and certified. Finding a naturopathic physician with a four-year degree and experience is another important step. Remember, naturopathic physicians can suggest a variety of options for your health plan and augment what you are doing with the GI clinic.

A few years ago, when my GI was adamant that I start 6MP and Remicade, I was despondent and scared. My naturopath said to look at it another way, that if a patient has no choice (given their quality of life), there could be other supplements and a range of beneficial treatments to help alleviate symptoms from the drugs. Many of us have no choice! We are lonely and confused, to say the least.

After sobbing on the kitchen floor after my recurrence in November of 2012, I picked up the phone and called Jessica Black, N.D. (a naturopathic doctor and my co-author of *Living with Crohn's & Colitis*) and asked for help. She recommended the curcumin-high-potency turmeric I now take daily (along with other supplements), and reassured me so I felt less overwhelmed. (I never did start the drug regimen, and remain in remission now for the second year!)

Not only did I get a second opinion from my naturopath, I also got one from a top Crohn's/colitis doctor at the famed Mayo Clinic in Rochester, Minnesota. My health insurance covered almost all of the cost for this (I just had to pay travel and lodging).

Being proactive about your diagnosis and the treatment plan presented to you, is a good way to stay involved in your own health and many naturopaths will work together with your clinic GI team for the betterment of your health. I highly recommend this approach, as it can help those in similar situations feel empowered and supported, with the goal of healing and leading a healthy lifestyle.

ELIMINATE STRESS IN YOUR LIFE

As many of us are aware, stress has a significant and impressionable influence on all diseases. In fact, stress and the hormones that are secreted in times of excess stress directly affect our health. In today's world, our lifestyles play a huge role in the prevalence of particular diseases, including all chronic illnesses and cancer.

Stress is a controversial cause of IBD because there are conflicting studies on the relation between stress and IBD. However, when we look at the picture of IBD through pathophysiology and clinical experience, it is clear that stress is absolutely connected to IBS. Stress may not be the *cause* of IBD, but it is certain that many with bowel disease report their symptoms and condition worsen when under stress.

If you have IBD and are reading this book, you can most certainly attest to what is being suggested. Haven't you spent more time in the bathroom when you are under extreme stress? Or before you have to give a presentation at work, or a lecture, or some other important event, do you ever feel "butterflies in your stomach," as the old saying goes?

Any chronic illness brings with it the complexities of the mind/body connection. Ways to de-stress in one's life can be easy, but like most things, require patience and practice. The following chapter will include a few tips to guide one who suffers from the myriad of symptoms related to IBD toward balance in their life. A few simple stress reduction techniques to consider are daily meditation and daily exercise, like walking or riding your bike. The Mayo Clinic recommends to start by identifying your stress triggers (for example work or family), and then take action to make positive changes. Daily life is stressful at times for everyone, but once you are aware of what causes your stress, you can find the key to successful stress reduction.

HOW TO MANAGE CROHN'S & COLITIS WHEN TRAVELING

We all get a wee bit revved up when a trip is on the horizon. For me, I also get anxious and fearful of having a flare-up on the road. I'm not alone, and I don't want you to feel alone either!

While travel is great, I have had numerous family vacations when my Crohn's flared up and left me in bed, throwing up and having to run to the bathroom. Needless to say, it was *not fun*.

About ten years ago, I was on a business trip at a printing press in Manitoba, Canada, and I was flaring up, and got a migraine on top of it. I was so embarrassed! I had to tell my client that I couldn't even do the press check I was paid to be doing!

To help you avoid situations like this, here are some tips for avoiding stress when you travel:

1. Eliminate stress that comes from secrets! Tell your travel companions you have IBD.
2. Rest every afternoon; go to bed early, walk on the beach...people will give you space.
3. *Carefully* watch what you eat when you travel. Avoid trigger foods! Pack a good supply of snacks that you know you can tolerate.
4. Drink lots of water.

Here is my travel kit of supplements:
- Grape seed oil extract
- Vitamin D
- L-Theanine (a calming extract of green tea, which helps with my anxiety about flying)

- My daily pills: phyto multivitamin, herbal adrenal assist, turmeric, magnesium-citrate, and Omega 3
- Ultra Flora™ Balance probiotics
- Echinacea and goldenseal (in case I catch a cold or get sick)
- Arnica gel and homeopathic Arnica tablets for sublingual use (in case I get injured—on a recent trip I whacked my knee and bruised it and the Arnica worked well)

STAY FOCUSED

In a recent study, *Mind Over Matter: Mental Training Increases Physical Strength,* by Erin M. Shackell and Lionel G. Standing from Bishop's University in Quebec, a group of college students were asked to imagine or visualize strength training versus a control group who did nothing and another group who did the actual physical work.

One area (hip flexing) was identified for groups of ten college student-athletes to work on for the two-week study. The ten college students who did the actual strength training five days a week did four sets of eight repetitions, adding five pounds of weight, and they saw strength training improvement of 28 percent. The group of ten that did nothing saw no gains; and the group that practiced visualization saw gains of 24 percent! This study was unique in that the group imagining themselves doing the reps actually did nothing after that—it was pure visualization.

The idea of using mental practice to improve performance has been around as long as Buddhism, which was founded 2,500 years ago. Exactly how visualization changes physical health remains a mystery, but the Dalai Lama spoke of the process of training the mind through meditation when I heard him speak at Middlebury College in 2012. I was profoundly affected by his talk. Those of us in the Crohn's-colitis community live with suffering sometimes on a daily basis, and it is important to develop and train your mind as a way to cope with it.

Additionally, studies have shown that altruistic behavior (the inherent, and possibly genetic ability to help) improves medical outcomes, so a good holistic lifestyle resolution could be: Do something kind for someone or something every day.

My own daily intention is this:

> *May our thoughts be kind and clear.*
> *May our words and communication be kind and clear.*
> *May our actions and intentions be for the greater good of all beings.*

I have used meditation and mindfulness steadily since my bowel resection six years ago, and I have made a daily practice of morning yoga and meditation. When I sit at the end of my yoga session (I use the gentle Rodney Yee DVD, *A.M. Yoga,*) I let his soothing voice guide me into a place where my breath slows, my mind quiets, and my shoulders and ears and limbs are relaxed. I chant "Om," before and after I sit, and I have a visualization that I let pass through my body from my head down through my spine, and out my lower back—it is a ball of white light. While this luminescent ball moves down my spine, I have a mantra I chant over and over that goes like this:

> *White light healing*
> *inflammation*
> *gone*

It is amazing to me how grounded and refreshed I feel after each morning session. I am sobered by the realization that the disease has been spreading back up my small intestine from the site of the surgery. However, I have heard from numerous health practitioners that a positive outlook actually affects disease outcomes, along with one's deepest hope for healing, so my goal is to be as upbeat as possible while I begin this naturopathic protocol. If you are just beginning this practice of meditation and setting healing and hopeful intentions, don't despair if you feel depressed or discouraged. It is incredibly helpful to sit and meditate, even if only for a few minutes each day. Many hospitals, like the Mayo Clinic, are including these techniques into their programs for patient care and disease prevention.

WATCH YOUR DIET

Start incorporating the dietary tips in Chapter 2 and begin keeping a daily food journal (see Chapter 4). It can also be helpful to be tested for allergens to find out if certain foods such as dairy or wheat are causing bloating or diarrhea.

Once you get in tune with your body, you can start to really tell whether certain foods make you begin to flare and you can back off immediately and note it in your journal to keep track. Also be sure to keep a list of safe foods and foods to avoid.

DIET AND WILLPOWER

My diet is very consistent, and I have maintained my weight of 139 pounds since I started taking control of my life, my disease, and my overall health. I kept a food journal for a year or so, beginning in 2006, and omitted wheat from my diet. The extra pounds stayed off, and I am healthier now than I was in my twenties and thirties (I am 55). Daily yoga (15–20 minutes with the Rodney Yee DVD, *A.M. Yoga*) and exercise (45 minutes a day, varying it, including walking, hiking, running, biking, yoga, tennis, etc.) help keep my weight consistent.

The question of willpower, for me, is almost a given: I follow a strict diet primarily eat food with just one ingredient, and have completely omitted refined sugar from my diet (I do use honey and a bit of maple syrup). Since most of the body's serotonin is produced by the enteric nervous system, I feel better emotionally, too. The Crohn's & Colitis Foundation of America (www.ccfa.org) has a good resource on their website. They even mention the SCD diet (see page 177), which I still use, in moderation.

Willpower can take many forms. For me, it is really a matter of focusing on getting well. When I used to diet to try to lose weight and achieve that ever-illusive American ideal of thinness, I never succeeded. My mind was focused on an ideal, and not on the practical day-to-day ritual of eating and exercising, and stretching with yoga. One way to achieve the kind of willpower you need is by writing in your food journal, and adding sections of motivational writing, or inspirational quotes from books or online sources. Plan a walk or dinner with friends and make it a challenge to cook gluten-free or grain-free. Most of all, don't be too hard on yourself and take it one day at a time.

EXERCISE DAILY

My rule of thumb for exercise is to keep it short, but keep at it. After my bowel resection, I would walk a few hundred yards each day; I gradually increased to my daily 4 miles. Start by getting out first thing in the morning after a cup of tea and try to climb some hills to get your heart rate up. Or follow a gentle yoga DVD (Rodney Yee's *A.M. Yoga* is wonderful) and set up a "yoga studio" in your house or apartment—find a spot that is peaceful and can become your own space.

Joining a walk or fundraiser can be a great way to get your exercise and also meet other IBDers, receive lifestyle support, make friends, and trade stories. Visit the Crohn's & Colitis Foundation of America (CCFA) for information on places to meet up for group walks or fundraisers. "Get Your Guts in Gear!" is the slogan for the annual walks for the CCFA, and they have these walks/fundraisers nationwide.

DEDE'S HOLISTIC HEALING TIPS

- Start keeping a daily food journal.
- Meditate daily.
- Walk 1–4 miles per day.
- Sleep at least 8 hours per night.
- Stay hydrated: drink water with freshly squeezed lemon or lime juice all day (carry a glass water bottle with you, some are now encased in non-breakable plastic or rubber for easy travel).
- Drink herbal teas—such as chamomile, dandelion root, or peppermint—and decaffeinated green tea.
- Before a shower, take a dry Loofa sponge and brush your skin all over, moving from the extremities toward your heart. Finish with a relaxing shower.
- Use essential oils daily (I like using lavender oil in my bath and eucalyptus oil in the shower).
- Massage your feet every night before you go to bed. Use a moisturizing lotion (with lavender, if you like). I also like to add organic apricot or sesame oil to make it thicker.
- Take Natural Calm magnesium powder by Natural Vitality each night in a hot glass of water before you go to bed to help you sleep better.

- Massage the back of your neck by pressing with acupressure in the "still point" at the base of your skull, or get a friend or spouse to help.
- Last, but not least, laugh every day! Watch those silly pet videos online, or call a family member or a friend with IBD, and swap funny stories.

BODY CARE

- Before a shower, take a dry Loofa sponge and brush your skin all over, moving from the extremities toward your heart. Finish with a relaxing shower.
- Use essential oils daily. (I like using lavender oil in my bath and eucalyptus oil in the shower.)
- Massage your feet every night before you go to bed. Use a moisturizing lotion (with lavender, if you like). I also like to add organic apricot or sesame oil to make it thicker.
- Take some Natural Calm magnesium powder by Natural Vitality each night in a hot glass of water before you go to bed to help you sleep better.
- Massage the back of your neck by pressing with acupressure in the "still point" at the base of your skull, or get a friend or spouse to help.
- Last, but not least, laugh every day! Watch those silly pet videos online, or call a family member or a friend with IBD, and swap funny stories.

Laughter is so important for emotional and physical health. In fact, researchers in Japan found laughter very effective in reducing inflammatory cytokines in rheumatoid arthritis patients. The same cytokines that were affected in this study are irregularly elevated in IBD patients. Therefore, we can make the assumption that laughter can affect inflammatory cytokines and may be an effective adjunctive therapy in the treatment of inflammatory bowel disorders.

Another study published in the *American Society of Hypertension Journal* supports that laughter coupled with yoga, which they term "laughter yoga", significantly reduced patient's diastolic and systolic blood pressure in addition to reducing patient's stress hormone, cortisol. Laughter yoga sounds fun!

So, armed with this cookbook, now is the time to set some goals for your health. Start your healthy diet and holistic healing changes, sign up for Team Challenge with the Crohn's and Colitis Foundation of America (www.ccfa.org), walk 3 miles a day (get your heart rate up by walking up hills), do yoga and meditate, get lots of sleep, and make an appointment with a local naturopath. Taking action, learning about your disease, and knowing how your body is affected will bring with it hope for new life.

CHAPTER 4

Keeping a Food Journal

WHEN YOU start out adjusting your diet and lifestyle to improve your symptoms, it can be immensely helpful to keep a daily journal—not just about the food you eat, but also what you do, how much you exercise and for how long, when you have acupuncture or massage, when you have your menstrual period (if you are a woman), or if you are exposed to anything potentially toxic in your environment—keep track of it all!

Jessica Black, N.D., says she has patients who immediately start making connections after starting a daily journal. (For example, you may notice right away that that whole bag of chips you ate the other day wasn't such a good idea.)

Take it slow, and modify your journal as necessary. Here are some modifications to keep in mind as you start examining your habits by looking at your daily journal:

1. See the change and believe in the change! Visualize optimal colon health daily. See yourself happy, active, and vibrant in your mind.

2. Proper mealtime habits: eat slowly, take your time preparing and shopping, and don't overeat.

3. Remove major dietary causes of inflammation: Keep a food journal, and stay away from trigger foods! (Often these trig-

ger foods are processed foods and fried or spicy foods, in addition to wheat, sugar, and dairy.)

4. Add only one supplement or herbal medicine, whichever best suits you. This may be an acute remedy for diarrhea, acidophilus, or any other supportive medicine. (For example, I started a new supplement called turmeric which is a natural anti-inflammatory. I take two capsules daily, and try to cook a curry dish once a week or so.)

5. Herbal teas: Pick one of the teas that best fit your needs and drink it daily. I drink peppermint. Also chamomile is a good stress reducer. Add honey for sweetening, as you like.

6. Take it slow and easy. Be kind to yourself, and ask for help!

As you now know, I balked at keeping a food journal when my surgeon first suggested it—I even made fun of it. However, it would have been helpful back in 2006 to have a plan. Using this cookbook and keeping your food journal will become a part of your path to healing and living with IBD. It should be easy and simple. I have made a list to help the transition, as follows:

- Figure out your healthy weight and get a complete physical from your naturopath. Make that appointment and get weighed, blood pressure checked, etc., and make a follow up appointment in a few weeks.

- Next, set a goal for your intention of journal keeping (once a day was my goal). Set up a time when you will log in, perhaps in the morning (to describe the day before), or at the end of the day.

- Note each time of day your cravings begin—especially useful at the beginning in the first few weeks—and do something to pamper yourself when that happens by making a smoothie, or having some tea with a bit of honey. A handful of nuts or trail mix (sugar-free, of course) can also help curb your appetite for sweet things.

- Create a summary of amounts, or cupfuls. It really helps

to pinpoint what may be upsetting your stomach. I finally figured out that coffee was the worst for me, and weaned myself to just ½ cup of coffee with ½ cup of added boiling water. This made a huge difference in helping me have regular bowel movements daily, usually in the morning, after breakfast. Too much coffee was obviously bad for my digestion, but I didn't admit it until I noted it in my food journal, and pinpointed the exact time of day.

- It is also a good plan to write down your reactions to stress. Note the time and date when things happen to you, or when you are feeling overwhelmed. Write a little note about it.
- Take note of any food reactions, too. Keeping a log like this will help you link your food to your mind, and by extension your food will become a part of your healing plan, like exercise and sleep, which should also be noted daily.

Before you know it, you will be writing your own book! Speaking of which, the idea of a journal connotes a dimestore variety spiral bound notepad, or traditional composition book, like the kinds you had at school. Whatever you use—iPad notes, dictated Siri notes on your smartphone or iPhone, writing on napkins and putting them all into a box in layers—it should be comfortable and ergonomically suited to your lifestyle. Get creative and most of all, be consistent and have fun with it.

CHAPTER 5

Shopping Tips for an IBD Diet

According to the Crohn's and Colitis Foundation of America, "There is no one single diet or eating plan that will do the trick for everyone with IBD. Dietary recommendations must be individualized. They should be tailored just for you—depending on which disease you have and what part of your intestine is affected."

Therefore, your shopping should be individualized as well. Here are some basic tips to get you started:

- To make it easy to follow your new diet, shop local and plan simple meals—most of us are busy and on-the-go, but with the new lifestyle plan and *Crohn's & Colitis Cookbook* for reference, you can budget and plan accordingly.
- Make a list: Plan a few meals for the week, like a delicious baked chicken or fish, a vegetable dish like a fresh pasta sauce with spaghetti squash instead of spaghetti.
- Buy locally raised and organic eggs and think about the small frequent meals when you make your list.
- Try to buy in bulk and bring your own bags and containers when you shop—many supermarkets now have organic and healthy food areas that also have bulk bins to save on packaging! Things to buy in bulk include honey, chamomile

and other tea, trail mix with walnuts, almonds, raisins, if you can tolerate it.

Breakfast: Buy enough ingredients for the week. Buy one melon, a few bananas, raisins, walnuts, almonds, cranberries, dried blueberries, gluten-free granola with no added sugar, almond milk (or whatever dairy-free alternative you like best that agrees with you), and some nice teas you can drink throughout the day—black tea is also okay, or half a cup of coffee (if you can tolerate it) with half boiling water. My one treat is to have a tablespoon of organic half-and-half in my tea in the morning.

Snacks: Trail mix of nuts and dried fruit (no sugar or chocolate), hard-boiled eggs, fresh-ground organic peanut or almond butter with fresh carrots, and different kinds of teas like green tea with mint or chamomile.

Lunch: Keep your lunches simple and fresh. Buy a nice fresh bag of organic lettuce (if you can tolerate salad), olive oil, balsamic vinegar, fresh local eggs, a few cans of tuna (dolphin-free and sustainably harvested), some healthy turkey from the deli, rice crackers or gluten-free bread, a bit of Canola oil mayonnaise, seedless organic mustard, carrots, and hummus.

Dinner: Again, keep your dinners simple. Buy organic chicken breast (sometimes I buy the precut, stir-fry kind), sustainably harvested fish (cod is easy to use, and non-farm-raised salmon is great), and lots of vegetables—plan your weekly veggie roast. Buy a spaghetti squash, if it is in season, for a pasta substitute; and always buy carrots, zucchini, onion, and pepper, along with lots of fresh garlic.

live; food that is not shipped from foreign countries, thereby losing nutritional value.

By shifting to an herb-friendly diet, the body will not only be receiving rich nutrients, but will also become more balanced as there are many herbs that actually calm the digestive track and soothe the process of elimination of the body's waste products. When herbs are introduced into a family's lifestyle through cooking, the benefits are myriad and rewarding in terms of health benefits, as well as social interaction. Cooking with herbs is a whole new way to utilize their health benefits and they taste good, too!

Increasing the intake of the right fruits, vegetables, grains, and meats while staying away from sugary and over-processed foods, can lead to better well-being. Some of the instructions for cooking and recipes in this book will also hopefully keep your health on track for years to come, and bring much joy into your life.

Remember that eating should be a pleasant experience, and eating well doesn't have to be a daunting task. Fresh herbs from your garden or a farmer's market; fruits and vegetables; lean, locally raised organic meats (or wild-caught and sustainably harvested fish); when eaten plain or in a delicious recipe, can brighten your day.

CUSTOMIZING THE RECIPES TO FIT YOUR NEEDS

It is important to remember that everyone is different, and your dietary needs will likely differ from those of someone else with IBD. Remember to consult your food journal frequently, and set goals for yourself. Perhaps you will go off wheat, dairy, and sugar for one month and see how you feel—most patients say they feel great after one month and many continue to be gluten-free, too. I ended up eliminating *all* grains and switched to a Paleo Diet that is sugar-free, grain-free, and dairy-free, and focuses on fruits, vegetables and animal protein.

Here are some helpful tips to keep in mind when creating recipes and creating a diet:

- All of the recipes in this book have been honed to be easy to re-create, with minimal ingredients needed. (I barely have enough energy as it is some days to pour myself a cup of water at the end of a day, let alone stand to cook for hours.) These recipes allow you more time to relax and less time to purchase a million ingredients. It's important to enjoy a meal that is delicious, and enjoy it without stress.

- Focus on the quality of food you put into your body. I try to buy organic and local as often as I can. Buying organic may not be feasible for all, so the "must" organic purchases should be meat and the Dirty Dozen (see page 61).

- Try to keep meals free from gluten, dairy, sugar, nightshades (eggplant, tomato, red pepper, and potato), red meat, and pork. The recipes in this book call for minimal grains while avoiding fried foods, processed foods, fast food, and anything artificial.

- Have fun! Not only is cooking fun, it can be part of your therapy. These recipes can be easily modified, so play with them and experiment until you find what works for you. Unfortunately, cooking for IBD does not fit a specific model. All diets are different and you should aim to explore new foods and see what works for you.

- Do not be too hard on yourself! Finding the diet and the recipes that work for you can be tough. There may be days when you "cheat"—I do it, we all do it. That is okay—just stand back up and try again. No one is perfect.

HOW TO PLAN YOUR MEALS

When it comes to healthy eating, planning ahead with shopping, and referring to the sample menus below will give you a good start in learning how to prepare healthy meals. You can mix and match meals, or substitute snack foods from the list on page 58. Don't be afraid to experiment and tailor the menus to your needs and preferences!

Here are some basic guidelines to follow when planning your daily meals:

- Eat breakfast.
- Eat a small amount of food every three hours.
- Eat a healthy meal at dinnertime.
- Eat a combination of vegetables and fruits.
- Eat healthy fiber, like rice-cakes, or a side-dish serving of rice.

This eating strategy gives you a steady, balanced stream of energy throughout your waking hours, for a total of approximately 1,200-1,500 calories per day.

SAMPLE MENUS

Breakfast

Scrambled egg or omelet with ¼ cup mushrooms, ½ cup spinach, and 1 tablespoon parmesan cheese (optional)
½ grapefruit
1 cup green tea

Mid-morning Snack Break

½ sliced apple with 2 teaspoons all-natural peanut butter

Lunch

1 rice cake, or romaine lettuce with 1 cup of tuna (use a natural, dolphin-free brand)

Mid-afternoon Snack Break

Veggies dipped into ½ cup hummus or olive oil and balsamic dressing

Dinner

Mixed green salad with red peppers and cucumber
Balsamic vinegar and olive oil
Broiled cod (scrod) with lemon pepper
3 ounces whole wheat angel hair pasta tossed with a bit of olive oil, lightly sprinkled with Parmesan cheese

Evening Snack Break

1 medium hard-boiled egg

Breakfast

Sugar-free natural muesli or wheat-free oatmeal
½ cup almond milk
1 cup dried raisins

Mid-morning Snack Break

10 almonds or 1 hard-boiled egg and three strawberries

Lunch

1 ounce fresh mozzarella, goat cheese, or avocado
1 sliced tomato on a bed of lettuce and basil, drizzled with olive oil and vinegar

Mid-afternoon Snack Break

Low-glycemic, 100-calorie protein bar
1 cup herbal tea, black

florets and dip into 2 ounces fat-free, sugar-free dressing of olive oil and balsamic vinegar

- 1 cup bean and chickpea salad: Toss diced celery, green pepper, cooked red beans, cooked chickpeas, and fresh parsley together with low-calorie balsamic vinaigrette
- ⅓ cup dry-curd cottage cheese with 4 olives and ½ medium tomato
- ½ cup low-fat cottage cheese with 5 strawberries
- For a special treat: 1 square 70% or higher dark chocolate with 5 almonds
- 1 whole hard- or soft-boiled egg
- Deviled egg: cut a hard-boiled egg in half, mix the yolk with hummus, and fill the egg
- 1 cup of soup (cream of tomato, cream of chicken, chicken noodle, or vegetable)
- 1 slice Wasa crispbread or rice cake with 1 ounce smoked salmon
- 1 slice whole grain bread (such as spelt) with 2 ounces fat-free turkey breast
- ½ cup couscous with celery sticks
- 1 cup fresh mango
- 1 cup cantaloupe
- 1 medium banana
- ½ cup grapes

THE DIRTY DOZEN AND THE CLEAN FIFTEEN

The Dirty Dozen is a guideline of twelve vegetables and fruits that typically contain the most pesticides of all the fruits and veggies out there. If you do decide to buy these fruits and veggies, it is recommended that you buy organic. I use this as my guideline when purchasing my vegetables and fruit.

The Dirty Dozen

Apples	Nectarines (imported)
Celery	Peaches
Cherry tomatoes	Potatoes
Cucumbers	Spinach
Grapes	Strawberries
Hot peppers	Sweet bell peppers

The Clean Fifteen

The Clean Fifteen is a list of fruits and veggies that tends to be safe, with minimal pesticides used on them.

Asparagus	Mangoes
Avocados	Mushrooms
Cabbage	Onions
Cantaloupe	Papayas
Sweet corn	Pineapples
Eggplant	Sweet peas (frozen)
Grapefruit	Sweet potatoes
Kiwi	

CHAPTER 7

Recipes

THE RECIPES in this book have been designed for cooks who still want to cook at home, but without the complex and time-consuming processes of the past. Let's face it: it is not realistic for most families to spend hours cooking in the kitchen every day. So, we have compiled this collection of recipes that are designed to be quick and simple while still remaining nutritiously tailored to the needs of IBD patients. We have included a few recipes for each category such as breakfasts, entrées, desserts, soups, and salads. Use what you learn from these recipes to begin developing your own. Everyone has different tastes and cultivating your palate takes time, patience, and sometimes trial and error. Learning to cook healthily is a process just like healing, so keep at it and stay positive.

Sarah Choueiry, who wrote the book's Foreword and contributed immeasurably to this cookbook, collaborated with me on the following recipes. She is the founder of the Crohn's Journey Foundation and is based in Los Angeles, but she and I are busy trading recipes and she has a wonderful recipe link on her website (see the Resources section). You can read about Sarah's own journey with Crohn's at the end of the book.

These recipes are meant to complement everything you have learned thus far about how to take care of yourself and how to live easily and healthfully with inflammatory bowel disease. In fact, this section is a part of your therapy in the process of healing your inflamed bowel. Remember, what you put into the gastrointestinal tract can have a direct effect on its functioning; therefore, nurturing it with nutrient-rich, anti-inflammatory foods sets the optimal foundation for healing.

However, you should keep in mind that not all recipes work for everyone. For example, some colitis or Crohn's patients may not be able to tolerate legumes due to extreme gas. Please consider what you can and cannot tolerate when planning your meals. These recipes are suggestions; feel free to substitute ingredients for your individual needs and tastes and for those of your family.

COOKING TO AID HEALING

When your body is healing, it needs easily digestible, nutritious foods to aid in the process. Additionally, the healing process requires adequate nutrients, especially easily digested protein. There is often inflammation associated with illness and/or recovery, so anti-inflammatory foods reduce swelling and inflammation and speed recovery. Enzymes are important to aid in digestion and to keep the flora in the digestive tract balanced. Choosing organic foods will decrease your toxin burden while your body is healing. The liver is responsible for producing many of the products necessary for healing. By eating foods lower in toxins and foods that support the liver, you will aid your body in recovery.

With the recipes in this book, we strove to offer "something for everyone," including those following a Paleo diet. In the following sections, each Paleo-friendly recipe has been indicated with a star.

Remedies for
When You Have
a Flare-Up

BEILER'S BROTH*

Ingredients:
   1 pound green beans
   2 pounds zucchini
   1 bunch regular parsley
   Filtered water, enough to cover all vegetables

Directions:
Bring vegetables to a low boil and continue to boil until very soft.
Strain the vegetables into a glass container and keep refrigerated.

WHAT IS MINDFUL EATING?

When approaching a meal, try to follow some simple mindful eating guidelines. For many of us, our bodies tend to be in a constant state of fight-or-flight, causing our cortisol levels to remain high, negatively impacting a lot of things in our bodies and throwing us out of whack. When adrenals are running high the blood meant to be in our digestive system is redirected to our limbs. When we experience stress and the blood supply in our guts is low, we do not digest food very well. This is where mindful eating comes into play. Here are four tips you can practice before approaching a meal to help reduce the stresses on your body, as well as being more present in your meal and allowing for better digestion. *How* you put food in your mouth is as important as *what* you put it in there.

1. Take five deep breaths before you begin your meal. Breathe in for four seconds, hold for two seconds, and then release for six seconds. It is a great way to reduce the level of stress in your body, especially if you are coming to a meal after a crazy work meeting, or running around with the little ones, or even frustrated from being sick all morning.
2. Put your fork or spoon down between bites. We don't realize it, but we tend to pile our food onto our fork and get it in our mouth before we have even finished swallowing what we have in our mouth already.
3. Chew well. This is helpful in so many ways; it slows down our eating and allows us to help out our digestive tract, aiding the stomach in breaking down food.

4. Eat slow. Really take your time to stop and smell the strawberries. Indulge in your meal, enjoy each bite and savor what you are eating. Make eating an experience, even if it is your twentieth bowl of soup in a row because your belly is just not up to handling solids just yet. Trust me: been there, done that—a positive state of mind can work wonders on your outlook.

Breakfast

BUCKWHEAT CREPES

Contributed by Sarah Choueiry
Ingredients:
  1 cup of buckwheat
  ½ cup flour rice
  ½ teaspoon salt
  1½ cups filtered water
  Coconut spray oil
  (Crepe pan needed for this recipe.)

Directions:
Mix all the ingredients in a medium bowl by hand. Cover the bowl and let it rest overnight in the fridge. The next day, generously spray a crepe pan with coconut spray oil and place on medium heat. Spoon enough crepe mix into the pan to cover the entire surface. Cook the crepe for about one minute, until it appears to almost cook all the way through. Flip it over for 15 seconds, then remove. Fill your crepes with your favorite fillings, or eat plain.

Tip: These crepes freeze well; just place parchment paper between each one before placing it in a freezer bag. Remove one at a time and warm in the microwave for 30 seconds.

BLUEBERRY SYRUP

This recipe was given to Dr. Black by Cathe Frederick.

Ingredients:

2 cups organic blueberries

Stevia, to taste

Directions:

Take two cups of blended blueberries and strain to remove seeds. Cook on low heat and stir frequently to form a light syrup. Cool slightly and sweeten with pure Stevia to taste. Serve over pancakes or light desserts.

EASY PANCAKES WITH GROUND PUMPKIN AND SUNFLOWER SEEDS

Ingredients:

3 tablespoons ground pumpkin seeds

3 tablespoons ground sunflower seeds

3 organic eggs

¼ cup non-gluten flour

¼ cup hemp milk, or other alternative milk

¼ cup uncooked millet (optional)

¼ cup blueberries (optional)

2 teaspoons baking soda

Directions:

Heat lightly oiled skillet to medium heat. Combine all ingredients except blueberries and millet into a medium-sized bowl and mix well until clumps have dissolved. Add blueberries and/or millet if you are going to use these ingredients. Pour batter into 3-inch diameter circles in the pan. When pancakes start to bubble, flip them carefully and cook on the other side until lightly browned on both sides.

OATMEAL FOR ONE

Ingredients:

- ⅓ cup gluten-free rolled oats
- ⅓ cup light coconut milk from a can (alternative: almond milk, rice milk, water)
- ⅓ cup water
- ¼ teaspoon cinnamon powder
- ½ teaspoon vanilla extract
- ½ organic banana, cut into thin slices
- Pinch of salt

Directions:

Place all the ingredients in a medium size pot and place on medium-low heat. Simmer for 7 to 10 minutes, stirring every minute. Once the oats have absorbed most of the liquids and gained a creamy consistency, it will be done. If you like it very creamy, add more coconut milk. Serve and eat immediately.

Tip: Use honey as an optional topping to make this dish a bit sweeter, and top with your favorite crushed nuts.

> I love eating oatmeal for breakfast. You can also cook this recipe in the microwave by placing all the ingredients in a bowl and heating it for 2 minutes. Cook longer if not at desired consistency. This is one of my go-to breakfasts that I take to work.

SMOOTHIE FOR ONE*

Contributed by Sarah Choueiry

Ingredients:

⅓ cup frozen organic blueberries

4–5 frozen organic strawberries

1 ripe organic banana

2 cubes of frozen dandelion, cilantro, and kale

1 hefty tablespoon of flaxseed powder

1 cup light coconut milk (water, almond milk, or plain rice milk)

½ cup filtered water

Directions:

Place all the ingredients in the blender and blend. I like to blend mine to a liquid consistency to insure that everything is broken down, allowing less work for my digestive system. If you like it thicker, go ahead and add ¾ of the liquids and add more from there until you get desired consistency.

I start every day with a smoothie. Any blender will do to make this smoothie. Once you get the hang of making the smoothie, you can begin to alter it to suite your taste buds and needs. If any of the fruits or vegetables I suggested bother you, don't add it or substitute something you find belly friendly for it. I juice 1 bunch of organic kale, 2 bunches of organic dandelion, and 2 bunches of organic cilantro at the beginning of each week and freeze them in ice cube trays. I use them throughout the week for my smoothies. All three have amazing anti-inflammatory properties.

For easy digestion and optimal absorption, blend the soup. This will break down the broccoli and carrots even further for ease of digestion. Taste and add tamari or sesame oil as desired for flavor.

The ingredients in this dish contain numerous benefits to a balanced gut. Elements like miso paste and tamari include helpful enzymes, while broccoli, carrots, and garlic contain important nutrients and boost liver health.

CURRY TURMERIC LEEK SOUP*

Ingredients:
   3 tablespoons olive oil
   2 leeks, sliced
   5 cloves elephant garlic, sliced into large slices
   ½ head Napa cabbage
   1 bok choy, chopped
   1 quart chicken broth
   1 can diced tomatoes
   3 teaspoons curry powder or more to taste
   1 teaspoon turmeric powder
   1 teaspoon fish sauce
   ½ teaspoon organic lemon juice
   Sea salt, to taste

Directions:
Add olive oil to large saucepan or soup pot on medium low heat. Add leeks and elephant garlic and sauté until medium soft. Increase heat to medium and add cabbage and bok choy and sauté for 3 to 5 minutes. Then add all other ingredients, cover, and simmer on medium to low heat until flavors mingle and vegetables are cooked but still maintain their crunch.

BUTTERNUT SQUASH SOUP*

Ingredients:

> 2 medium butternut squash, peeled, halved, seeded, and cubed
>
> 1 cup sweet onion, chopped
>
> 1 teaspoon fresh ginger, grated
>
> Approximately ¼ cup maple syrup
>
> ¼ teaspoon ground nutmeg
>
> ¼ teaspoon ground cinnamon
>
> ¼ teaspoon ground cardamom
>
> 4½ cups homemade chicken stock
>
> Coarse salt and freshly ground pepper, to taste
>
> ¼ cup heavy cream (optional)
>
> 1 tablespoon new fresh chives or parsley (optional)

Directions:

Steam the squash. Fry onion and ginger and add the spices and chicken stock when the onions are translucent. Blend everything in a blender and serve hot, garnished with either chives or parsley. The soup may be stored and refrigerated for up to three days, or frozen for long as two months.

GRANDMA'S CHICKEN SOUP

Contributed by Sarah Choueiry
Serves about 3–4 people
Ingredients:

> ½ organic chicken
>
> Cinnamon stick (about 6 inches length)
>
> 1 dried bay leaf
>
> 1 lemon (optional)
>
> Salt, to taste (approximately 2 teaspoons)

Directions:

Place the half chicken in a medium pot and add enough water to cover it by ½ an inch. Turn the heat on medium-high and bring it to a boil. As it is coming to a boil, take a ladle to skim impurities and fat that rise to the top. Do this until the water appears clear. Add the bay leaf, cinnamon and salt, cover. Reduce to a simmer and cook for 75 minutes. Once it is done, remove the chicken and the cinnamon stick. Taste to see if you need to add more salt and enjoy your delicious, organic clear broth.

For added variety, try some variations on the broth. Add a handful of washed, rinse rice to the broth and simmer for an additional 15 minutes. Once done, take a hand blender and blend it all together. Add diced carrots and half a diced yam to the broth and simmer for an additional 20 minutes, until soft, and add shredded chicken. *

Tip: I like to squeeze half a lemon into my bowl but only do that if you can handle the acidity.

I lived off this soup while hospitalized in September 2012, and for 3 months afterwards once I got home. I loved this soup because it grew with me and became more complex as my diet expanded. I initially just had the broth for a week (my family ate a lot of chicken that week). Then, my grandma would add rice to it and blend it to thicken up the soup for me. Once I gained more strength, I was able to add some shredded pieces of chicken and some carrots and sweet potato pieces. This is one of the soups I still revert to when I have had a bad food reaction or a flare up. I hope this soothes your insides, as it has mine.

LENTIL APRICOT SOUP

This soup was introduced to Dr. Black by her good friend, Desiree LeFave, a licensed midwife.

Ingredients:

   3 tablespoons olive oil

   1 onion, chopped

   2 cloves garlic, minced

   ⅓ cup dried apricots, minced

   1½ cups red lentils

   5 cups vegetable broth or chicken broth

   ½ teaspoon ground cumin

   ½ teaspoon dried thyme

   3 plum tomatoes, peeled, seeded and chopped 2 tablespoons fresh lemon juice

   Salt, to taste

   Ground black pepper, to taste

Directions:

Sauté onion, garlic, and apricots in olive oil. Add lentils and stock. Bring to a boil, then add spices, reduce heat, and simmer for 30 minutes, covered and stirring occasionally. Add tomatoes and simmer 10 minutes more. Add lemon juice and puree half of the soup in the blender. Add pureed half back into the remaining soup and serve warm.

LENTIL SOUP

Makes 12 cups

Ingredients:

   1 pound brown lentils

   Water

   ¼ pound salt pork

   ½ cup onion, chopped

   1 cup celery and leaves, chopped

   ½ cup carrots, chopped

   1 clove garlic, chopped

   1 bay leaf, crumbled

   1 teaspoon honey

   ¼ teaspoon thyme leaves

   2 tablespoons butter

   2 tablespoons flour

   1 tablespoon lemon juice

   Scallions, thinly sliced

Directions:

Wash lentils. Soak overnight in enough water to cover the lentils. Drain soaking water and measure. Add additional water to make 2½ quarts. Combine lentils, measured water, and salt pork in soup pot. Bring to a boil. Reduce heat and simmer for 2½ hours. Add chopped vegetables, garlic, bay leaf, honey, and thyme. Simmer for another 1 to 1½ hours.

Remove salt pork from soup pot and put in blender jar with a cup of soup liquid. Blend until smooth. Return to soup pot. In another pan, add butter and blend in flour. Add 2 cups of hot soup to flour mixture and bring to a boil, stirring constantly. Return to soup and stir in lemon juice. Heat to serving temperature and season to taste with salt. Serve garnished with sliced scallions.

FRESH MINESTRONE SOUP*

Serves 4

Ingredients:

- 1 onion, chopped
- 1 garlic clove, crushed
- Pinch oregano
- 1 teaspoon margarine, melted
- 1 small potato, peeled and diced
- 1 carrot, diced
- ¼ pound green beans, diced
- 1 stalk celery
- 1 small tomato
- Some parsley, chopped
- 1 small leek (optional)
- ½ can mushrooms (optional)
- ½ cup corn (optional)
- 2 okras, cut (optional)
- ½ cup zucchini, sliced (optional)
- ¼ cup cabbage, shredded (optional)

Directions:

Combine onion, garlic, and oregano with margarine. Cook over low heat until onion is golden. Add 2 cups water and bring to a boil. Add vegetables with the firmest added first. Simmer on low heat until vegetables are tender, but still crisp. Serve in warm soup bowls, thickly garnished with parsley.

COLD CUCUMBER SOUP*

Serves 6–8

Ingredients:

3 large cucumbers

½ onion, sliced thin

2 tablespoons butter, unsalted

½ cup bay leaves

1 tablespoon white rice flour

3 cups low-sodium, fat-free chicken broth

1 teaspoon kosher salt

1 cup almond milk, unsweetened

2 tablespoons lemon juice, fresh or bottled

½ teaspoon dill weed, fresh or dried

1½–2 cups dairy-free sour cream

Additional dill (for garnish)

Directions:

Peel two of the cucumbers. Slice and sauté cucumbers in butter along with the onions and bay leaves until tender, but not brown. Blend in the flour. Add broth stirring until smooth. Add salt and simmer covered for 25 minutes. Discard bay leaves.

Puree in food processor or blender. Pour through a strainer and discard any solids. Chill well. (The soup can be frozen at this point, or refrigerated for up to 2 days.) The day of serving; skim off any fat on the surface. Add almond milk, lemon juice, and dill weed to the chilled mixture. Peel the remaining cucumber; cut it in half length wise, scoop out the seeds, and coarsely grate. Cover and refrigerate until serving time. This can be done 1–2 hours ahead.

Place about 1 heaping tablespoon of grated cucumber in the bottom of each bowl. Add soup and a dollop of sour cream.

FARMERS' MARKET SOUP*

Serves 6

Ingredients:

Stock

    1 medium carrot, minced

    1 stalk celery, minced

    2 medium onions, minced

    1 medium shallot, minced

    1 medium leek, minced

    3 cloves garlic, crushed and unpeeled

    7 cups homemade chicken broth (or use low-sodium canned broth)

    6 peppercorns

    1 sprig fresh thyme

    5 parsley stems

    Nonstick spray

Soup

    2 medium leeks, white and light green parts only, halved lengthwise and cut into 1-inch lengths

    6 small red potatoes, scrubbed, cut into ¾-inch chunks

    1 cup frozen peas, thawed

    2 cups packed baby spinach

    2 tablespoons chopped fresh parsley leaves

    1 tablespoon chopped fresh tarragon leaves

    Salt and fresh ground black pepper, to taste

Directions:

Stock

Completely wash and clean all vegetables used in stock (and soup). Combine the carrot, celery, onions, shallot, leek, and garlic in a heavy-bottomed stock pot. Lightly spray the vegetables with cooking spray, toss, and coat. Cover and cook the vegetables over medium heat, stirring until slightly softened and translucent, about 6 minutes. Add the broth, peppercorns, thyme, and parsley stems. Increase the heat to medium high and bring to a simmer. Continue until stock is flavorful (about 15 minutes). Strain the stock, discarding solids.

Soup
Bring the stock to a simmer in a large heavy pot over medium heat. Add the prepared leeks and potatoes and simmer until potatoes are tender, about 9 minutes. Stir in peas, spinach, parsley, and tarragon. Season to taste with salt and pepper.

EXCELLENT SAVORY TOFU STEW

Serves 6–8
Ingredients:
    ¼ cup olive or vegetable oil
    3 onions, thinly sliced
    4 carrots, thinly sliced
    4–5 stalks celery, thinly sliced
    2–3 cloves garlic, minced or pressed
    1 cup firm tofu (press out excess water)
    1 ½ cups zucchini or yellow squash, ¼-inch slices
    2 fresh tomatoes, diced
    1 tablespoon dried basil
    2 bay leaves
    2 cups tomato juice
    ⅓ cup soy sauce (or tamari)

Directions:
Heat oil in a large lidded pot over medium heat. Add onion, carrots, celery, and garlic, cooking until onions are transparent. Add tofu, zucchini or squash, and tomatoes. Simmer a bit, and then add herbs.

Simmer for 2–3 minutes. Pour in tomato juice and soy sauce; stir. Reduce heat to low, cover pot, and simmer for one hour.

JULIE'S PISTOU

Serves 4

Ingredients:

1 tablespoon butter

1 medium onion, diced

1 leek, diced

2 large tomatoes, peeled, seeded, and crushed

4 cups chicken or vegetarian stock or water

½ pound fresh green beans

3 potatoes, cut into bite-sized pieces

Approximately ¼ pound of spaghetti, broken in half

2 cloves garlic, crushed

Several basil leaves, crushed

2 tablespoons olive oil

2–3 tablespoons broth (chicken or vegetarian)

4 tablespoons Parmesan cheese, grated

Salt and pepper, to taste

Directions:

In a medium heavy pot over medium-low heat, melt butter and slowly cook onion and leek. Add tomatoes. Add stock or water to pot and bring to a boil. Add fresh green beans and potatoes. Season with salt and pepper, to taste. When vegetables are almost cooked (about 15 minutes) add spaghetti. Reduce heat and finish cooking very slowly.

While cooking, to make the pesto, pound the garlic with several basil leaves. Add, while still pounding, olive oil and 2–3 tablespoons chicken or vegetarian broth. Serve soup, dividing pesto and Parmesan cheese between portions.

White beans, zucchini, and carrots can all be added; if you are in a hurry, cheat and use already prepared basil pesto.

Another childhood favorite, this was always a late summer or early harvest meal based on what was in the garden.

Salads and Side Dishes

༄

ARUGULA, AVOCADO AND CUCUMBER SALAD*

Contributed by Sarah Choueiry
Serves 3–4 people
Ingredients:
Dressing
    ½ teaspoon salt
    2 tablespoons balsamic vinegar
    3 tablespoons extra virgin olive oil
    ¼ teaspoon garlic powder
Salad
    2 large handfuls of organic baby arugula
    3 organic, Persian cucumbers, peeled and diced
    1 ripe organic avocado, diced

Directions:
Place all the dressing ingredients in a jar and shake. Clean the vegetables then place the vegetables in a medium bowl and toss with as much dressing as you would like. *

KALE AND CARROT SALAD
Ingredients:
Salad
> 1 bunch kale, chopped
> 5 large carrots, sliced
> 2 tablespoons sesame seeds
> 2 tablespoons hemp seeds
> Sea salt, to taste

Dressing
> 1 tablespoon sesame oil
> 1 tablespoon olive oil
> ⅓ cup brown rice vinegar
> 1 teaspoon pure maple syrup

Directions:
Steam carrots and kale until soft, but still crunchy and let cool. Mix with seeds, coat with dressing mixture, and store in the refrigerator. Flavors will mix if left overnight. Serve chilled.

Tip: If seeds like sesame or hemp cause digestive problems, omit them from the recipe or do not make this recipe. I also recommend grinding the seeds first (a coffee grinder works well).

EASY SALMON SALAD*
Ingredients:
> 2 cans wild boneless, skinless salmon
> ½ cup mayonnaise, organic
> ½ cup minced carrots
> ½ cup minced apples
> ¼ cup sweet relish, organic and sweetened naturally

Directions:
Mix all ingredients in a large bowl. Serve chilled with crackers, as a salad, or alone.

SPINACH SALAD

Serves 4

Ingredients:

Dressing

- 2 tablespoons olive oil
- 1 tablespoon cider vinegar
- 1 tablespoon chopped fresh parsley
- 1 teaspoon lemon juice
- ¼ teaspoon maple syrup

Salad

- 1 cup cooked rice noodles
- 2 cups torn raw spinach or salad mix
- ¾ cup sliced celery
- ¼ cup sliced green onions
- 1 medium tomato or 1 cup cherry tomatoes
- ½ cup raw snow peas
- 1 cup seedless grapes (optional)
- ½ pound cooked shrimp or 8-ounce chicken breast (optional)

Directions:

Place all dressing ingredients in pint jar, close with lid, and shake well. Cook noodles according to package directions, but do not add salt to water. Drain, rinse, and cool. Place torn fresh spinach in large salad bowl. Chop celery and green onions. Slice fresh tomato into small wedges or cut cherry tomatoes into halves. Wash grapes (if using) and snow peas and add all to salad bowl.

If using cooked fresh or frozen shrimp, remove peels and veins. If using cooked chicken, cut into bite-size pieces using separate cutting board. Add to salad bowl. Place drained and cooled pasta in salad bowl. Shake dressing and pour over salad. Toss with salad tongs or two large spoons. *(if you omit rice noodles)*

CHICKPEA SALAD WITH LEMON AND PARMESAN

Serves 2

Ingredients:

1 (15-ounce) can chickpeas, drained and rinsed

1 teaspoon fresh lemon juice

1½ teaspoon olive oil

¼ cup loosely packed shredded Parmigianino Reggiano, or dairy-free substitute

1–2 finely minced garlic cloves (optional)

Pinch of salt

Directions:

Combine all ingredients in a bowl, and stir gently to mix. Taste, and adjust seasoning as necessary. Serve immediately, or chill, covered, until serving.

This little salad only has five ingredients, so make sure that they're all of good quality. There's no room for second-rate pantry closet cast-offs here, so don't even think about it! First of all, be sure to use a good brand of chickpeas. Also, get out your best olive oil—one you'd want to eat from a spoon, if you're into that sort of thing. This salad keeps well in the fridge and is, in my humble opinion, best eaten cold.

WARM SALMON SALAD AND CRISPY POTATOES

Serves 4

Ingredients:

- 2 tablespoons extra virgin olive oil, divided
- 2 small yellow-fleshed potatoes, scrubbed and cut into ⅛-inch slices
- ½ teaspoon salt, divided
- 1 medium shallot, thinly sliced
- 2 teaspoons rice vinegar
- ¼ cup buttermilk
- 2 (7-ounce) cans boneless, skinless salmon, drained
- 4 cups arugula

Directions:

Heat 1 tablespoon of olive oil in a large nonstick skillet over medium-high heat. Add potatoes and cook, turning once, until brown and crispy (5–6 minutes per side). Transfer to a plate and season with ¼ teaspoon salt; cover with foil to keep warm. Combine the remaining 1 tablespoon oil, ¼ teaspoon salt, shallot, and vinegar in a small saucepan. Bring to a boil over medium heat. Remove from heat and whisk in buttermilk. Place salmon in a medium bowl and toss with the warm dressing. Divide arugula among four plates and top with the potatoes and salmon.

HIPPY YUM-YUM SALAD*

Serves 4

Ingredients:

- 1 red onion
- ⅓ cup chives
- 1 medium-sized red potato
- ½ large sweet potato

⅓ cup olive oil
Pinch of fresh rosemary
2 medium heads of romaine lettuce
2 shredded, sliced or peeled carrots
1 avocado
½ cup hummus (see page113)
⅓ cup balsamic vinegar
Pinch of fresh dill
Juice of half a lemon

Directions:
Cut up onion, chives, and the two potatoes (very thinly sliced). Dump olive oil in a large frying pan. Put in onion, potato, chives, and rosemary into frying pan. Stir occasionally.

Cut up romaine lettuce, carrots, and avocado into a bowl. When frying pan ingredients have browned and are sizzling, dump them in with the salad. Pour in balsamic vinegar and mix with hummus and lemon juice, and sprinkle with dill.

Salmon, sardines, chicken, or chickpeas can be added for protein.

CARROT, APPLE, AND RAISIN SALAD*

Serves 8
Ingredients:
    1 large (8-ounce) apple, peeled and cored
    2 teaspoons lemon juice
    ¾ pound raw carrots
    3 tablespoons dark raisins
    ⅓ cup dairy-free sour cream

3 tablespoons almond or coconut milk

1 teaspoon maple syrup

¼ teaspoon ground cinnamon

¼ teaspoon ground nutmeg

Directions:

Peel, core, and shred apple. Place apple in large mixing bowl and toss with lemon juice. Peel and grate carrots. Toss carrots and raisins with apple. Mix non-fat sour cream with milk, sweetener, cinnamon, and nutmeg in small bowl. Pour over carrot mixture, toss with rubber scraper to coat; divide into serving bowls. Cover tightly with plastic wrap and chill for 1 hour or more.

For preparing in food processor:

Fit food processor with metal chopping blade. Place non-fat sour cream, milk, lemon juice, sweetener, cinnamon, and nutmeg in bowl of food processor. Blend on and off to mix. Unplug food processor and remove metal chopping blade, leaving sour cream mixture in bottom of mixing bowl. Fit food processor with grating tool. Grate carrots and apples directly into sour cream mixture. Turn off food processor and remove grating tool. Turn mixture into serving bowl. Sprinkle raisins over top of mixture and toss to blend.

Cover tightly with plastic wrap. Chill 1 hour or more before serving.

CRISPY BAKED BRUSSELS WITH CARROTS*

Contributed by Sarah Choueiry

Serves 4

Ingredients:

> 1 pound whole Brussels sprouts (approximately 1 16-ounce bag), cut into quarters

2 cups (about 4–5 medium sized) carrots, peeled and sliced
    fairly thin
⅓ cup extra virgin olive oil
¾ teaspoon salt
½ teaspoon garlic powder
¼ teaspoon pepper
Juice of half a lemon

Directions:
Preheat oven to 400°F. Mix all of all of the ingredients *except* the
lemon in a bowl. Place the mixed ingredients onto a foiled baking
(cookie) sheet and spread out evenly. Bake for 20 minutes, then take
a look and toss around the Brussels sprouts and carrots, turning them
over if browning has begun on the bottom. Rotate the baking sheet;
some ovens have more heat in the back then in the front and we
want to distribute the heat evenly. Cook for an additional 10 minutes.
Remove the baking sheet and squeeze on the juice of half a lemon on
top of the Brussels sprouts and carrots. Lightly toss and serve.

ALMOND CHEESE SPREAD

Contributed by Sarah Choueiry
Ingredients:
    1½ cups almond meal
    ¼ fresh lemon juice
    ¼ cup extra virgin olive oil
    1 garlic clove minced
    ¼ teaspoon of thyme
    ½ cup water

Directions:
Add all of the ingredients to a food processor and blend for 5 minutes. Line a strainer with a couple of layers of cheesecloth, pour the

mixture into the cheesecloth and collect the ends of the cloth and tie together, making a little sack. Leave the cheese in the strainer, place the strainer on a plate and refrigerate overnight.

The next day, preheat the oven to 350°F. Generously spray a small oven safe bowl with non-stick spray. Gently remove the cheese from the cheesecloth and place in the bowl. Bake the almond spread for 40 minutes until lightly brown on the top. Remove it from the oven and let it cool.

Serve with your favorite gluten-free crackers or spread on a brown rice tortilla. This dish will last about a week in the fridge.

> This is another of my mom's recipes. I am blessed to have a creative mom, and because I miss cheese at times, she decided to create a "cheese" I can eat. This one is a bit more time consuming, but makes for a fun activity to do on a weekend.

TABOULI*

Ingredients:
- 1 cup quinoa, cooked and cooled
- 2 bunches of parsley, regular or flat leaf, minced
- 1 pint cherry tomatoes, cut in fours
- 2–3 cloves garlic, chopped fine
- ½ cup organic lemon juice
- ⅓ cup organic cold pressed olive oil
- Sea salt, to taste

Directions:

Start by cooking the quinoa. Add 1 cup of quinoa and 2 cups filtered water to a pan and cover. Bring to boil, reduce heat to medium low and allow it to come to a boil/simmer, until all the water has been absorbed. Stir occasionally to keep the quinoa from burning on the bottom of the pan.

When all the water has been absorbed, remove from heat and allow to cool. Add cooked quinoa, parsley, garlic, and tomatoes into a large bowl. Pour lemon juice, olive oil and salt over the mixture. Mix well and chill in refrigerator for at least 30 minutes prior to serving. Chilling for at least 24 hours helps the flavors mingle even better.

This makes a very pretty dish and always a great dish to bring to a potluck or celebration meal. If you cannot tolerate tomatoes, try replacing them with chopped cucumbers and Kalamata olives.

GREEN DRINK

Ingredients:
  1 bunch parsley
  2–3 cups filtered water
  Lemon juice concentrate, to taste
  Molasses, to taste

Directions:

Blend ingredients on high in a blender until it reaches a smooth consistency. It will be frothy, but will reduce as it sits. Drink chilled.

This is an everyday drink for some of Dr. Black's patients. If you want to use this drink therapeutically, it will cleanse your colon and your blood. Make this drink and drink of its yield daily for 3 days in a row; on the fourth day, make a new drink. That way, you will only need to make the drink about two times per week. If you have sensitive digestion, or if raw foods bother you, begin by drinking only small amounts to gauge your tolerance to the large amount of raw fiber.

CRISPY YAM FRIES

Contributed by Sarah Choueiry

Serves 2

Ingredients:

1 hannah yam

¼ teaspoon salt

¼ teaspoon ground black pepper

¼ teaspoon garlic powder

¼ cup extra virgin olive oil

Nonstick spray (I prefer coconut oil spray)

Directions:

Preheat the oven, 400°F. Cut the yam into thin fries, about ¼ inch width and height, 3–3.5 inches in length. Place a piece of foil on a baking sheet and spray the foil with non- stick spray. Place the cut up yam fries into a bowl and toss with the olive oil.

Mix the salt, pepper, and garlic powder in a small bowl. Evenly spread the oiled fries on the baking sheet and evenly sprinkle on top with about 3/4 of the spice mix. *

Bake for 15 minutes and flip the fries over and rotate the baking sheet in the oven. Cook for an additional 5 minutes and check on them, bake until lightly golden brown. Every oven is different, so keep an eye on them for the last couple minutes to insure you don't burn them. Taste to see if you want to add any additional seasoning, and serve.

BEST ROASTED VEGGIES

Adapted from Molly Watson's recipe, Local Foods (localfoods.about.com)

Making roasted vegetables is as easy as putting them in the oven, but making the *best* roasted vegetables—soft and tender, browned and caramelized, full of intensified flavor—involves a few tricks. Make roasted vegetables as delicious as possible by following the ten tips below:

1. Preheat the Oven
This is an important step. You want the oven nice and hot when you go to put the vegetables in. A less-than-hot oven will turn out less-than-browned vegetables. The exact temperature doesn't matter too much. I tend to set the oven to 375°F, but anything in the 350°F to 425°F range will work.

2. Cut Vegetables into Even Pieces
Smaller vegetables can be roasted whole, as long as they are of even sizes. You want even pieces so the vegetables cook at an even rate. In general, vegetables need to be trimmed and cut—larger pieces will make a more dramatic presentation whereas smaller, bite-size pieces are easier to eat.

3. Toss Vegetables with Oil

In a roasting pan or a large bowl, toss vegetables with 1–2 tablespoons or two of olive oil or the oil of your choice. Oil helps the vegetables brown, so don't skip this step. Drizzle vegetables with the oil, then toss them to coat as evenly as possible. You can add coarsely chopped garlic, slices of chilies or pepper flakes, or other seasonings at this point, too.

4. Don't Crowd the Vegetables

You want plenty of hot air to be surrounding the vegetables. The less the vegetables touch each other, the more area on them will brown.

5. Sprinkle Vegetables with Salt

The reason roasted vegetables at restaurants always taste so great is that they are seasoned in stages. A bit of salt at the beginning, and another small dose of salt when they're done. Give the vegetables a sprinkle of salt before you pop them in the oven. You can give a final sprinkle of salt at the end, so just add a little bit here.

6. Roast Vegetables at the Top

Roasting the vegetables in the top third of the oven will help the vegetables brown the best.

7. Shake or Turn Vegetables

When the vegetables start to brown, give the pan a good shake, or else use a spatula to turn the vegetables to move them around a bit to brown evenly.

8. Roast Vegetables Thoroughly

You want roasted vegetables to be two things: brown and tender. Keep the vegetables in a hot oven until they are both. If they start to get too dark, cover them with foil until tender, and then cook for a final 5 minutes or so with the foil off. If they aren't browning, raise the heat in the oven and move the pan to the top of the oven.

9. "Finish" the Vegetables
Roasted vegetables are best with a final drizzle of good quality olive oil and a little sprinkle of salt. Other final hints of flavor can include:

- Freshly ground black pepper
- Fresh lemon juice
- Minced herbs (mint, parsley, thyme, or just a wee bit of rosemary are great choices)
- Balsamic vinegar

10. Serve Vegetables Warm or Let Them Cool
Roasted vegetables are great while still warm, obviously, but they can also be served at room temperature to great effect. If you want to serve room-temperature roasted vegetables, however, be sure to let them cool in a single layer, uncovered or else very loosely covered, so that the vegetables don't start to steam each other.

ROASTED AUTUMN VEGGIES*

Serves 4
Ingredients:
Olive oil
1 onion, cut in half and sliced in thin crescents
1 sweet potato/yam, peeled, cubed
12 small carrots, sliced in circles
6 Brussels sprouts, cut off ends and cut in half or quarters
Kosher salt, to taste

Directions:
Preheat oven to 350°F. Mix all the veggies together in a medium glass baking dish that has been coated with olive oil. Toss with a spoon and extra olive oil to, lightly coat. Add kosher salt, and toss some more.

Bake for 40 minutes or until soft when pricked with a fork. Make sure the veggies are soft enough for easy digestion. Don't use Brussels sprouts if they cause a reaction. Can use zucchini or peppers, or other seasonal veggies.

STEVE'S RAWSOME GUACAMOLE*

Ingredients:
2 large avocados (or 3 small ones)
Juice of 2 limes (about ¼ cup)
1 medium tomato (or 2 Roma tomatoes), chopped
¾ cup fresh cilantro, chopped
⅓ cup green onion, chopped
1 teaspoon minced jalapeño pepper (red or green)
1 teaspoon sea salt

Directions:
Put the avocado flesh into a bowl. Add the lime juice. Mash the avocado and lime juice together with a fork until creamy. Fold in tomato, cilantro, green onion, jalapeño pepper, and sea salt. Enjoy!

This guacamole works especially well as a dip for organic carrot and celery sticks. It also goes well with flaxseed crackers. If you aren't a raw foodist, it goes well with tortilla chips, too. Feel free to adjust the ingredient ratios to suit your tastes (i.e., more green onion, more jalapeño, more or less salt, etc). If you like spicy guaca- mole, feel free to double or triple the jalapeño (or more). The version above is pretty mild. Guacamole is one of my favorite foods, so I'd like to share my best guacamole recipe that I got from my friend, Steve. I tweak this recipe every time I make it (thanks to my daughter, Emma).

HUMMUS

Serves 6–8

Ingredients:

    2 cups chickpeas, drained and well cooked or canned (cooking liquid reserved, if possible)

    ½ cup tahini

    ¼ cup extra virgin olive oil (plus oil, for garnish)

    2 cloves garlic, peeled (or to taste)

    Juice of 1 lemon (plus more as needed)

    Salt and freshly ground black pepper, to taste

    1 tablespoon ground cumin or paprika, or to taste (plus a sprin- kling for garnish)

    Fresh parsley leaves, chopped (for garnish)

Directions:

Put the chickpeas, tahini, oil, garlic, and lemon juice in a food pro- cessor (or a blender for even smoother hummus), sprinkle with salt and pepper, and begin to process; add chickpea-cooking liquid or water as needed to produce a smooth puree. Taste and adjust sea- soning, adding more salt, pepper, or lemon juice as needed. Serve, drizzled with some olive oil and sprinkled with a bit of cumin or paprika and some parsley.

FAVORITE STEAMED CARROTS*

Serves 4

Ingredients:

   5–6 carrots, scrubbed with a brush under cold running water (if
      not organic, you should peel them)
   1 tablespoon brown sugar
   Canola margarine

Directions:

Melt margarine in a saucepan under medium heat. Add carrots and
sauté until tender (about 5–10 minutes). Add brown sugar and sauté
a bit more. Serve as a delicious side dish, hot or cold.

You can make this dish even healthier if you steam the
carrots first and then quickly add them to the frying pan.

GRASSO'S SAUTÉED KALE*

Serves 6

Ingredients:

   2 large bunches fresh kale (preferably from your garden)
   1 large red onion
   4 cloves garlic, minced
   4 tablespoons olive oil
   1 tablespoon balsamic vinegar
   1 tablespoon water

Directions:

Rinse kale bunches. Chop the leaf portion loosely, and cut the stems
into ½-inch lengths.

Leave the kale in a colander in your sink while you prepare the other ingredients. (Note: you can sprinkle with lemon juice before-hand to further enhance the beneficial phytonutrients found in this vegetable; in fact, I always have lemon in my kitchen to sprinkle on fresh fruits and vegetables while I cook. It not only enhances the benefits but also keeps them from turning brown).

Preheat large cast-iron frying pan with olive oil. Add garlic and sauté quickly until the garlic turns a tan color. Add chopped red onion and sauté a few more minutes. Add the chopped kale (it may seem like a lot of kale, but don't worry; it will shrink down quickly, so you can add it in batches if your skillet is too small) and stir briskly as it cooks, coating the kale in the oil-garlic-onion mix. Once the kale is darker and turning limp, add the balsamic vinegar and stir, quickly adding the water, and cover to steam the whole dish (the kale absorbs the flavors in this way).

Serve hot as a side dish for most any meal. Kids love this dish, too, and kale is widely recognized as being a great detoxification food and one of the healthiest of vegetables. One thing to note: the way I like to cook kale, via my friend Tom Grasso, is not "quite" as healthy as steaming, during which the fiber undergoes some beneficial binding, but it is just so delicious cooked this way and it is still beneficial.

Seafood Entrées

✑

GARLIC-HERBED SCALLOPS*

Serves 4

Ingredients:

2 tablespoons unsalted butter

2 tablespoons cream extra virgin olive oil

2 garlic cloves, thinly sliced

1 teaspoon lemon zest

2 teaspoons fresh lemon juice

2 teaspoons chopped fresh oregano

2 teaspoons chopped fresh tarragon

1 pound sea scallops, rinsed and patted dry (approximately 8)

Directions:

Coat the grill rack with nonstick cooking olive oil. Preheat grill to high for the sauce, and install a small saucepan. Heat butter and olive oil over medium heat until butter melts. Add garlic and cook, stirring until just softened. Remove from heat. Spoon 3 tablespoons of the garlic mixture into a small bowl. Add lemon zest, lemon juice, oregano, tarragon; and salt and pepper to taste. Cover and set aside.

Place remaining garlic mixture in a medium bowl. Add scallops, and salt and pepper to taste; toss to coat. Grill covered for 2–3 minutes per side, or until scallops are opaque in the center. Transfer scallops to a serving platter, drizzle with sauce, and serve.

LEMON STEAMED FISH*

Serves 2

Ingredients:

½ pound cod, halibut, or scrod fillets (or other mild white fish)
2 tablespoons onion, finely chopped
2 tablespoons fresh parsley, finely chopped
½ teaspoon dill weed
⅛ teaspoon paprika
1 teaspoon lemon juice
Dash of pepper

Directions:

Preheat oven to 375°F. Center each fillet on a 12-inch square of foil. Sprinkle with onion, parsley, dill weed, paprika, pepper, and lemon juice. Fold foil over fillet to make a packet and pleat the seams to securely enclose the packet. Place on cookie sheet and bake for 30 minutes.

> This recipe is easy to prepare, with little clean-up required. It is also low in fat and carbohydrates.

ALMOND CRUSTED FISH*

Serves 2

Ingredients:

½ pound mild, white fish fillets (sole, flounder, orange roughy, etc.)

⅙ cup sliced almonds

1 tablespoon reduced-fat margarine, melted

1 tablespoon lemon or lime juice

½ teaspoon Worcestershire sauce, low-sodium

¼ teaspoon paprika

⅛ teaspoon pepper

Nonstick spray

Directions:

Preheat oven to 375°F. Coat pan with cooking spray. Rinse and pat fish dry, arrange in pan in a single layer. In a small bowl, mix almonds, margarine, lemon or lime juice, Worcestershire sauce, paprika, and pepper. Top fillets with the above mixture and spread evenly. Bake 12–15 minutes or until the fish flakes easily.

STEVE'S FISH*

Serves 2

Ingredients:

1½ pounds wild, fresh-caught pollock

½ cup dry white wine

3 small tomatoes

1 small onion

12 black Tuscan olives, with pits

1 teaspoon olive oil or canola margarine

Parmesan cheese, to taste

Directions:
Preheat oven to 350°F. Wash and dry fish and place in a glass baking dish. Pour white wine over the fish. Cut up tomatoes (in chunks) and onions (in half-moon slices) and arrange over the top of the fish. Add black olives here and there, as desired. Add olive oil to sprinkle over the top. Cover with aluminum foil and bake for 20 minutes.

Check to see that the fish is done by flaking it with a fork. Bake uncovered for a bit more time. Before serving, sprinkle some freshly grated Parmesan cheese over the top.

> This recipe works well with a tossed salad of romaine lettuce, red peppers sliced thin, sliced carrots, and avocado. A side dish of roasted vegetables is also perfect with this delicious and savory fish recipe that my husband makes for our happy household.

BAKED SCALLOPS

Serves 4
Ingredients:
    1 pound fresh scallops
    ½ cup half-and-half
    ½ cup white wine
    2 tablespoons butter
    1 cup seasoned breadcrumbs, gluten-free

Directions:
Preheat oven to 375°F. Cover scallops with half-and-half in a greased casserole dish. Add a splash of white wine. Dab with pats of butter. Sprinkle liberally with seasoned breadcrumbs. Cover and bake for 45 minutes.

FISH CURRY

Serves 4

Ingredients:

- 2 tablespoons butter
- 3 onions, chopped
- 2 cloves garlic, peeled and crushed
- 3 tablespoons parsley, chopped
- 1½ teaspoons turmeric
- 1 teaspoon salt
- 1½ tablespoons coconut
- 1 ½ teaspoons curry
- 3 tomatoes, cut into wedges
- 3 tablespoons yogurt
- 1½ pounds scrod, cut into small pieces

Directions:

Heat oil, and sauté onions, garlic, and parsley until onions are lightly browned. Add turmeric, salt, coconut, and curry. Mix well. Cook for 3 minutes at medium heat.

Add tomatoes and cook for 10 minutes. Stir in yogurt and cook for 5 minutes over medium heat. Add fish, cover well with sauce and let curry come to a boil. Cover and simmer for 10 minutes.

BAKED SALMON*

Contributed by Sarah Choueiry
Serves 2
Ingredients:
    1½ tablespoons extra virgin olive oil
    About 1 pound salmon filet, cut into two pieces
    ½ teaspoon salt
    ½ teaspoon pepper, or to taste
    ¼ teaspoon garlic powder
    ¼ teaspoon cumin powder
    1½ tablespoons extra virgin olive oil
    1 lemon

Directions:
Preheat the oven to 400°F. Place 1 ½ tablespoons of olive oil on a small foil covered rimmed baking sheet. Place the salmon on the baking sheet, skin side down. Evenly sprinkle both fillets with salt, pepper, garlic powder, and cumin. Place in the oven for 10 minutes.

Remove and let it sit for 5 minutes. The fish continues to cook a little once out of the oven. Squeeze a half a lemon on top of both fillets. Take the other lemon half and cut into wedges to serve with the salmon.

This dish is a go-to meal in our house; not only is it easy to digest but it's filled with those Omega-3s that you want in your body to help reduce inflammation.

BROILED MARINATED FISH*

Serves 4

Ingredients:

    2–4 pounds fish

    2 teaspoons powdered cumin

    1 clove garlic, crushed

    Juice of ½ lemon

    1 teaspoon dried savory, crushed

    1 cup soy sauce

    1 tablespoon olive oil

Directions:

Rinse fish and pat dry. Cut three diagonal slashes about 1½ inch apart with a sharp, thin-bladed knife. Place fish in a shallow baking dish and combine all remaining ingredients.

Pour mixture over the fish on each side and marinate in the refrigerator for 4 hours. Preheat broiler for 10 minutes. Remove fish from marinade and lightly pat dry. Broil 10 minutes on each side, basting twice with marinade.

CONNIE'S GRILLED SALMON*

Serves 4

Ingredients:

- 1 pound wild salmon fillet
- 2 tablespoons olive oil (1 tablespoon for seasoning plus 1 table-spoon for ginger sauce)
- Juice from 1 lemon (1 tablespoon for seasoning plus 1 tablespoon for ginger sauce)

Ginger Sauce

- 1 tablespoon lemon juice
- 1 tablespoon olive oil
- 1 clove garlic, minced
- 2 tablespoons grated ginger
- ½ teaspoon soy sauce
- 2 tablespoons chopped cilantro
- 1 teaspoon Dijon mustard
- Salt and pepper, to taste

Directions:

Season fillet with a dash of lemon juice, pepper, and olive oil. Place on a pre-heated grill and cook salmon 6–8 minutes per side. Brush on sauce and serve. Serve with new red potatoes and tarragon butter (mix soft butter with chopped tarragon).

Meat and Poultry Entrées

BAKED CHICKEN WINGS*

Contributed by Sarah Choueiry
Serves 4
Ingredients:
  1½ pounds chicken wings
  2 tablespoons extra virgin olive oil
  1 teaspoon salt
  ½ teaspoon garlic powder
  ½ teaspoon ground pepper
  Wing sauce (your choice)

Directions:
Preheat the oven to 400°F. Wash the chicken wings and pat dry. Remove the tips from the chicken wings and separate the wings at the joint. Toss the wing parts with the olive oil, salt, pepper, and garlic powder. Arrange the chicken on a sprayed, foil-covered, rimmed baking sheet. Bake for 25 minutes and turn wings over.

Bake for an additional 10 minutes. Place under the broiler for 2–3 minutes, keeping an eye on it the whole time to insure you do not burn it but get that perfect golden crispy skin on the wings. Toss in your dressing of choice. I prefer them plain or tossed with a little Paleo barbecue sauce for some flavor.

ROASTED CHICKEN*

Adapted from Bobby Dern
Serves 4
Ingredients:

- 2 pounds broccoli, cut up into florets, and some stems
- 2 tablespoons olive oil
- 1 tablespoon organic chicken broth
- 2 garlic clothes, chopped
- ½ teaspoon ground cumin
- 1 teaspoon of salt, or to taste
- Fresh ground black pepper, to taste
- Hot chili powder, to taste
- 1 pound organic, boneless, skinless chicken breasts, cut into chunks
- Finely grated lemon zest, to taste
- Lemon wedges (for garnish)

Directions:

Preheat the oven to 425°F. In a baking pan combine the broccoli, 1 tablespoon of oil, the broth, half the garlic, the cumin, the salt and pepper, and the chili powder. Toss the ingredients to coat, and then spread the broccoli out in a single layer. Roast for 10 minutes.

In a large mixing bowl, combine the chicken and lemon zest, remaining 1 tablespoon oil, and the remaining garlic with salt and pepper. Toss the ingredients. Take out the baking sheet the baking pan from the oven, add the chicken, and toss together with the broccoli. Return the baking pan to the oven and roast, tossing once or twice halfway through the cooking time, until the chicken is cooked through and the broccoli is tender and golden around the edges, not much longer than 10 minutes. Take the lemon wedges and add them to the plate.

GROUND TURKEY AND VEGGIE LENTIL SAUTÉ

Serves 4

Ingredients:

- 1 pound ground turkey
- 1½ teaspoons sea salt
- 1 tablespoon cumin
- 1 tablespoon oregano
- 3 medium zucchini, sliced into rounds
- 10 ounces fresh or frozen corn
- 1 (28-ounce) cans chopped tomatoes, undrained
- 1 cup steamed, cooked lentils

Directions:

Brown ground turkey in a large skillet and season with salt, cumin and oregano. Add sliced zucchini and corn, and continue to cook until tender. Add tomatoes and lentils, reduce heat to low, and simmer 10 minutes. Taste and adjust seasoning to your liking.

CHICKEN STIR FRY*

Ingredients:

- 1 pound organic chicken breast slices
- 2 small cloves of garlic, chopped
- 2 tablespoons wheat-free tamari
- 1 teaspoon of fresh ginger, grated
- Salt and pepper, to taste

Directions:

Mix the above ingredients in a small bowl. Let the mixture stand in order to marinate, for about 20 minutes. If you don't have enough time you can cook it right away. Place cooking oil in pan; once it is heated, add chicken and sauté, stirring constantly until done.

BAKED CHICKEN IN TWO EASY STEPS*

Serves 4
Ingredients:
  3–4 pounds chicken, cut into 8 parts (2 breasts, 2 thighs, 2 legs,
    2 wings)
  Olive oil
  Salt and freshly ground pepper, to taste

Directions:
Preheat the oven to 400°F. Rinse chicken pieces in water and pat
dry with paper towels. Coat the bottom of a roasting pan with olive
oil. Rub some olive oil over all of the chicken pieces in the roasting
pan. Sprinkle both sides of the chicken pieces with salt and freshly
ground black pepper. Arrange the pieces skin-side up in the roasting
pan so the largest pieces are in the center (the breasts) and there is
a little room between pieces, so that they aren't crowded in the pan.
    Cook for 30 minutes at 400°F. Then lower the heat to 350°F and
cook for 10–30 minutes more (approximately 14–15 minutes per
pound total cooking time). Continue until juices run clear (not pink)
when poked with a sharp knife, or the internal temperature of the
chicken breasts is 165°F and the thighs 170°. If your chicken pieces
aren't browning to your satisfaction, you can put them under the
broiler for the last 5 minutes of cooking, until browned sufficiently.

CHICKEN AND RICE

Contributed by Sarah Choueiry
Serves 4
Ingredients:
  1 tablespoon organic grass-fed butter
  2 tablespoons extra virgin olive oil
  2 organic chicken breasts, bone in, skin on, washed and patted
    dry

2 organic chicken legs, washed and patted dry2 teaspoons salt

½ teaspoon ground pepper

1 teaspoon ground allspice

⅛ teaspoon powdered cinnamon

5–6 cups filtered water

2 cups of Calrose rice (or short grain rice)

Directions:

Place the butter and olive oil in a large pot, under a medium heat. Let the butter melt and cook for 1–2 minutes, until the oil and butter begin to slightly sizzle. Place the chicken breasts and legs in the pot, skin side down, for 5 minutes. Sprinkle ½ teaspoon salt, ¼ teaspoon pepper, and ½ teaspoon allspice on top of the chicken. Once the skin achieves a golden brown color, turn it over to brown the other side, about 5 minutes. Sprinkle ½ teaspoon salt, ¼ teaspoon ground pepper, ½ teaspoon allspice, and the ground cinnamon.

Once all sides are browned, add 5–6 cups of filtered water, until the chicken is almost all covered. Turn up the heat to medium-high and bring to a boil. Once it has reached a boil, add ½ teaspoon salt, cover and bring it to a simmer on a low heat for 75 minutes. Place your rice in a medium-size bowl and fill the bowl with filtered water, about an inch or two above the rice and set that aside.

Once the chicken is done, remove it and set aside on a plate to shred once it has cooled. Reserve chicken broth. Rinse the rice well under cold running water a couple of times and strain. In a medium pot, add 2 cups of the chicken broth and the pre-soaked rice. Add ½ teaspoon of salt; taste the broth to see if you feel it is needed. Bring it to a boil, cover, and simmer for 10 minutes exactly. Shred the chicken as the rice is cooking. Once the rice is done, do not open the cover; just set aside for 5 minutes. After 5 minutes, place the shredded chicken on top and enjoy!

This was one of my favorite dishes growing up. I use 1 tablespoon of organic, grass-fed butter in this dish because I know that it won't bother me. If butter does not settle well in your system, eliminate it and heat oil on a medium-low heat. You can also substitute vegan butter for the butter. I love this dish with a side of my arugula, avocado, and cucumber salad. You will also have leftover broth; you can save that in the freezer and take it out on a night you want to make some flavor filled rice.

COCONUT CURRY CHICKEN OVER BROWN RICE

Ingredients:

    3–4 chicken breasts

    2 cups water

    1–2 vegetable bouillon cubes, sodium-free

    2 cups rice, cooked

    3 tablespoons olive oil

    1 onion, chopped

    3 large carrots, sliced

    ½ head of cabbage, chopped

    2 broccoli florets, chopped

    1 teaspoon turmeric powder

    2 teaspoons curry powder, or more to taste

    1 bag frozen organic peas

    1 can coconut milk

    1 tablespoon fish sauce

    Filtered water, to taste

    Sea salt, to taste

Directions:

Prepare chicken breasts by putting them in a Crock-Pot in the morning with bouillon cubes mixed with 2 cups of water. Cook on low all day.

When preparing dinner, begin by cooking the rice. Add rice and 2 cups filtered water to a pan. Bring to boil and boil for 1 minute while stirring, then cover and reduce heat to low. Let simmer for about 10 minutes, or until rice has absorbed the water.

Bring olive oil to medium-low heat in a large sautéing pan or wok. Add onion and sauté until soft and translucent. Increase heat to medium and add carrots, cabbage, broccoli, turmeric, and curry powder and sauté until the color in the vegetables is more vibrant. Use a fork to pull the chicken meat away in the Crock-Pot until it is shredded. Add entire contents of the Crock-Pot and frozen peas to the sautéed vegetables and keep stirring. Reduce heat to low-medium and add fish sauce, salt, and coconut milk and continue to cook until flavors mingle but vegetables are still crisp. Serve over cooked brown rice.

> This chicken curry requires a little preparation because the chicken is cooked in a Crock-Pot all day prior to the dinner preparation.

EASY MARINADE FOR CHICKEN, SALMON, OR TOFU

Ingredients:
  2 parts wheat-free tamari
  1 part honey
  1 part dark sesame oil
  1 teaspoon grated ginger
  1 clove minced garlic

Directions:
Mix all ingredients together. Coat salmon, chicken, or tofu and allow it to sit overnight before preparing.

BUFFALO STEAK MARINATED IN TEQUILA, LIME, AND SALT*

This recipe was inspired by Dr. Black's friend and amazing cook, Rosalinda Camacho in Lafayette, Oregon.
Ingredients:
  2 pound buffalo steak
  ½ cup tequila
  3 tablespoons lime juice
  1 teaspoon sea salt

Directions:
Add steak and all other ingredients to a small dish or Ziploc® bag. Rotate often for 24 hours and grill or cook to medium-rare.

LAMB SHEPHERD'S PIE

Serves 8
Ingredients:

Mashed Potatoes
  6 medium Yukon gold potatoes, peeled and chopped
  2 tablespoons butter, softened
  ⅓ cup cream
  1 egg
  1 tablespoon olive oil
Meat Mixture
  2 tablespoons olive oil
  1½ pounds ground lamb

½ medium yellow onion, peeled and chopped

4 garlic cloves, peeled and thinly sliced

½ large red pepper, chopped

2 cups button mushrooms, quartered

1 cup carrots, peeled and chopped

1 teaspoon dried lavender

2 teaspoons dried rosemary

½ cup red wine

2 cups chicken stock

2 tablespoons cornstarch

2 tablespoons water

Directions:

Potatoes

Set a large saucepan filled with cold water over high heat. Add enough salt to the water to make it taste like the ocean. Add the potatoes. Bring to a boil, and then reduce the heat to medium-high. Simmer until you can slide a knife right through one of the potato pieces without any force, 10–15 minutes.

Pour the potatoes into a large colander and shake to make sure all the water is out. Let the colander sit in the sink for 3–4 minutes to steam the potatoes dry. If you own a potato ricer or food mill, push the potatoes through. Or, you can push the potatoes through a fine-mesh sieve with the back of a ramekin or ladle.

Put the potatoes back into the pot you cooked them in. Stir the softened butter into the potatoes. Add the cream, egg, and olive oil and stir with a rubber spatula until the potato puree is silky smooth.

Meat

Set a large skillet over medium-high heat. Pour in the oil, and then add the ground lamb. Cook, stirring occasionally, until the lamb is thoroughly browned. Remove from the pan and set aside.

Add the onions to the pan in which you cooked the lamb, along with the garlic. Cook until the onions are soft and translucent, stirring frequently (about 5 minutes). Add the pepper, mushrooms, and carrots and cook until the carrots are softened, about (5 minutes). Add the lavender and rosemary and cook until they release their fragrance (about 1 minute). Add the meat back to the vegetable mixture and remove from heat.

Pour in the red wine. Cook, stirring occasionally, until the wine has reduced by half its volume. Add the chicken stock and bring it to a boil. Combine the cornstarch and water and stir until you have a thick slurry. After the chicken stock has simmered for a moment, pour in the slurry and stir the mixture thoroughly. This will thicken the liquid into gravy.

Turn on the oven to broil. Transfer the meat and vegetable mixture to a large pie pan. Top with the potato puree. Cook under the broiler until the potatoes have turned a dark golden-brown (about 10 minutes). Serve immediately.

BEEF STEW*

Ingredients:

Braised Beef
   5 pounds boneless beef chuck (not lean), cut into 2-inch pieces
   3 tablespoons olive oil
   3 carrots, quartered
   3 celery ribs, quartered
   2 medium onions, quartered
   1 head garlic, halved crosswise
   3 tablespoons tomato paste
   ⅓ cup balsamic vinegar
   1 (750 ml) bottle dry red wine (about 3 ¾ cups)
   2 Turkish bay leaves or 1 California bay leaf
   2 thyme sprigs

3 cups reduced-sodium beef broth

3 cups water

Vegetables

2½ pounds small white boiling potatoes

1½ pounds carrots, peeled and sliced into thin rounds

Directions:

Preheat oven to 350°F with rack in middle. Pat beef dry and season with 2 ½ teaspoons salt and 1 teaspoon pepper. Heat oil in pot over medium-high heat until it shimmers, then brown meat, without crowding, in 3 batches, turning, about 8 minutes per batch. Transfer to a platter. Reduce heat to medium, and then add carrots, celery, onions, and garlic and cook, stirring occasionally, until well browned, about 12 minutes.

Push vegetables to one side of pot. Add tomato paste to cleared area and cook paste, stirring, 2 minutes, then stir into vegetables. Add vinegar and cook, stirring, 2 minutes.

Stir in wine, bay leaves, and thyme and boil until wine is reduced by about two-thirds, 10–12 minutes.

Add broth to pot along with water, beef, and any juices from platter and bring to a simmer. Cover and braise in oven until meat is very tender, about 2½ hours.

Set a large colander in a large bowl. Pour stew into colander. Return pieces of meat to pot, and then discard remaining solids. Let cooking liquid stand 10 minutes.

While beef braises, peel potatoes and cut into 1/2-inch-wide wedges. Slice carrots diagonally (1-inch). Add potatoes and carrots to stew (make sure they are submerged) and simmer, uncovered, stirring occasionally, until potatoes and carrots are tender, about 40 minutes.

SAVORY RACK OF LAMB*

Contributed by Sarah Choueiry
Serves 4

Ingredients:

1 teaspoon salt
½ teaspoon black pepper
½ teaspoon garlic powder
1 (8-rib) Frenched racks of lamb (each rack 1½ pounds), trimmed
   of all but a thin layer of fat
Coconut oil spray (for pan)

Directions:

Mix together the pepper, salt and garlic powder in a small bowl. Cut the rack of lamb into 8 individual ribs. Place a piece of plastic wrap on top of the ribs and pound the meat to about half the original size.

Place your pan over medium heat and spray generously with coconut oil. Let the pan heat up for about 3 minutes, coconut oil is a great oil to use because it tolerates high heat before burning. Place the ribs, four at a time to not crowd the frying pan, and season generously with a quarter of the spice mix. Let it cook for about 3 minutes and then turn over for 2 more minutes. Season again with a quarter of the spice mix. Remove after two minutes for medium to medium-well done. Spray the pan again with coconut oil and repeat with the last four pieces of lamb.

I love lamb. I can digest it well and it just tastes so good. I get teased because I eat it to the bone. Enjoy with some baked yam fries, with the arugula salad, or a side of baked Brussels sprouts with carrots.

ALMOND "BREADED" TURKEY CUTLETS*

Contributed by Sarah Choueiry

Ingredients:

¼ cup plus 1 tablespoon coconut flour

1¼ teaspoon salt

1 teaspoon ground garlic powder

¾ teaspoon ground black pepper

¼ teaspoon paprika (optional)

1¼ pounds turkey breast cutlets, about 6–7 pieces

3 eggs

1¼ cups almond meal (almond flour)

4 teaspoons organic coconut oil

Directions:

Get three shallow plates and set them up for your assembly line. Mix the coconut flour, ¼ teaspoon salt, ¼ teaspoon garlic powder, and ¼ teaspoon pepper on one plate. Crack 3 eggs and whisk in the second plate. Mix the almond flour, 1 teaspoon salt, 1 teaspoon garlic powder, ¼ teaspoon paprika and ½ teaspoon ground black pepper in the last plate.

Take your turkey cutlets and place them between two pieces of plastic wrap and pound until ¼ inch in width.

Set up your station by putting two forks in each dish. Use the forks from the coconut flour plate and grab your first turkey cutlet. Place the turkey cutlet in the flour mixture, coating all sides of the turkey with flour. Remove and shake any extra flour off. We want it to be lightly dusted. Place it in the egg mixture and coat both sides with egg, lift off and allow excess egg to drip off before placing in the almond mixture. Place in the almond mixture, making sure all sides are coated. Place the breaded turkey on a parchment paper lined baking tray and set aside. Repeat the steps with each turkey cutlet until all are breaded.

Heat up a nonstick pan on a medium heat with 1 teaspoon organic coconut oil for about 2 minutes. Cook two turkey cutlets at a time and let them sit on one side first for 3 minutes, and then flip once you see a nice golden brown crust forming. Let them cook for an additional 2–3 minutes on the other side, until cooked through. They will not take long to cook. Taste one to see if you would like to add more salt; if yes, just sprinkle some on top as you remove them. Place them on an iron rack to allow them to cook without softening the bottom. For every batch you make add in another teaspoon of coconut oil into the pan.

Enjoy with a side salad, some of our yam French fries, or take as a snack on the go. If you do not have an iron rack, you can take one of the racks directly out of your oven and use that. Place foil underneath and set it on the kitchen counter. You can also "bread" half of them and place them in freezer bags and place in freezer to cook at a later time. Great for those days you work late and want something quick to cook. Let it defrost on the counter for at least 30 minutes and follow instructions above to cook!

> I love anything breaded and fried, but being gluten-free and avoiding fried foods makes it a bit tough to indulge. I hope you enjoy it as much as I do.

LEMON BAKED CHICKEN BREASTS*
Contributed by Sarah Choueiry

Ingredients:
Chicken Breasts
   3 pounds chicken breasts (approximately 6 chicken breasts)
   ¼ cup extra virgin olive oil
   ¾ teaspoon ground black pepper
   1 teaspoon salt

Yam Mixture:

> 1–2 Hannah yams (or potatoes) cut into roughly ½ inch cubes, around 5–6 cups
>
> 1 teaspoon salt
>
> ⅛ cup extra virgin olive oil
>
> ⅓ teaspoon ground black pepper
>
> Juice of 2–3 lemons (about ½ cup) mixed with 2 tablespoons of water

Directions:

Wash the chicken breasts and pat dry. Place the chicken breasts in a deep baking dish, making sure they do not go on top of each other but can be touching. Drizzle half the olive oil on one side and sprinkle on top half the pepper and salt. Turn over the chicken and pour the remainder of the olive oil and sprinkle the remainder of the salt and pepper. Let the chicken marinate in the olive oil, salt, and pepper while the oven preheats. Place the chicken in the oven, uncovered for 20 minutes. Flip the chicken over and cook for another 20 minutes, uncovered.

Mix all of the yam mixture ingredients together in a bowl and spread on top of the chicken. Tightly cover the tray with foil and place back in the oven for 30 minutes. Check the potatoes; if they are soft to the touch, they are ready to go onto the next step. If they are not, cook, covered, until tender. Take it out and let it cool for 5–10 minutes. Add the lemon juice with water mixture and place back under the broiler, uncovered, for about 10 minutes, until the potatoes get a nice, light-brown crisp on top.

> This is a great dish when you have guests coming over and you want to impress them but still eat something you can enjoy. It is a bit time consuming but not hard and well worth it. You can also cut the recipe in half if you are not planning to feed so many people.

GARLIC GINGER CHICKEN PATTIES*

Contributed by Sarah Choueiry
Serves 10–12
Ingredients:

    1½ pounds of ground, organic chicken (or turkey)

    1 tablespoon grated ginger

    3 cloves of crushed garlic

    1 tablespoon lemon juice

    1 teaspoon salt

    ½ teaspoon pepper (optional)

    Coconut oil spray (or 2 teaspoons coconut oil)

Directions:

Mix all the ingredients together except the coconut oil. Don't "over-work" the ground chicken, or it will get tough. Make patties with your hand, pressing lightly to make them thin, and place them onto a plate. Your patties should be about 4 inches in diameter and ½ inch thick. Place 1 tablespoon of coconut oil in a fry pan over medium-high heat. Add 3–4 patties at a time, do not overcrowd. Cook on each side for 2–3 minutes.

Repeat steps 3 and 4 until you have cooked all your patties. This is a great dish to enjoy with my cucumber, avocado and arugula salad.

To freeze for another day: Stack about 3–4 raw patties on top of each other, placing a piece of parchment paper between each patty. Place in a freezer bag and freeze. When ready to cook, just remove the bag from the freezer and let it sit on the counter for 1–2 hours to defrost, or place in the refrigerator the night before and cook the next day. To cook, follow the instructions above.

> My mom and I came up with this recipe when I was still healing from my hospitalization and wanted to eat something with more flavor. If any of the ingredients do not settle well for you, omit them.

STEVE'S CHICKEN-MARENGO*

Serves 4

Ingredients:

 1 chicken (2–3 pounds), cut
 2 tablespoons olive oil
 1 clove garlic, minced
 5 green onions (scallions), minced
 ½ cup white wine
 ¼ teaspoon thyme
 ¼ cup tomato sauce
 1 tablespoon parsley
 Salt and pepper, to taste

Directions:

In a large heavy skillet, brown chicken in olive oil until golden. Remove pieces to a warm bowl; salt and pepper to taste. Add onions and garlic to skillet and heat until transparent and golden. Add wine, thyme, and tomato sauce to skillet, scraping bottom; heat until bubbly. Add chicken; cover and cook at 350°F for 30 minutes on stove. Garnish with parsley.

CONNIE'S GRILLED VEGGIES AND TURKEY BURGERS

Serves 4–6

Ingredients:

Marinade

 ¼ cup olive oil
 Juice of one lemon
 Splash of balsamic vinegar
 A few shakes of pepper

Vegetables
1 zucchini, sliced lengthwise, ¼-inch thick
2 red, green, orange, or yellow peppers, sliced
3/4 red onion, thickly sliced
1 bunch asparagus, sliced
7–8 mushrooms, sliced (optional)

Turkey Burgers
2½ pounds lean, ground turkey
1 pound crumbled gorgonzola
⅓ cup red onion, chopped
3 cloves garlic, peeled and crushed with garlic press

Bread
1 pound pan rustque, or all-natural flatbread

Directions:
Turkey Burgers
Mix all the burger ingredients together and form into patties.

Vegetables
Put vegetables all in a Ziploc® bag with marinade and shake it up, then refrigerate for at least one hour. Arrange vegetables on a pre-heated grill and grill on moderate heat, covering the grill for first 5–10 minutes. Start to turn vegetables over and repeat as necessary (black grill lines are one indication of doneness). When vegetables are almost done, put the burgers on and cook next to vegetables

Bread (omit if grain-free):
Slice bread thickly and brush inside with olive oil. Towards the end of cooking, add the bread slices to the edges of the grill and heat up on both sides. Serve on platters, family-style.

Vegetable Entrées

JULES'S SUMMER SAUCE FOR PASTA

Serves 4

Ingredients:

- 6 ripe medium-size tomatoes, finely chopped
- 2 cups (8 ounces) sliced mushrooms
- 6–8 ounces mozzarella cheese (fresh mozzarella is best), shredded or grated
- ½ cup chopped fresh basil
- 2 garlic gloves, minced
- ½ cup olive oil
- 1 teaspoon salt
- 1 pound spaghetti or linguine
- ½ cup Pecorino Romano cheese

Directions:

Mix all ingredients, except pasta and cheese, together in a bowl and let stand for 1 hour at room temperature. Cook pasta; drain. Pour sauce on hot noodles and sprinkle with cheese.

GLUTEN-FREE TEMPURA VEGETABLES

Serves 6

Ingredients:

Tempura

  2 cups rice flour (or mix of coconut flour and almond flour)

  1 teaspoon baking soda

  1 teaspoon garlic powder

  ¼ teaspoon sea salt

  2 cups cold carbonated water

  Your choice of vegetables (see below)

Tentsuyu Dipping Sauce

  ¼ cup gluten-free vegetable stock (or dashi if you have it)

  1 tablespoon maple syrup

  ¼ cup gluten-free tamari

  1 tablespoon rice vinegar

  ¼ cup water

Directions:

Tempura

Preheat vegetable or olive oil in a deep pan to approximately 300°F. Combine the dry ingredients in a medium-size mixing bowl. Add the carbonated water and whisk until smooth. Lightly dip ingredients in the batter and immediately fry them until crispy. It takes longer to fry vegetables than to fry seafood. Drain Tempura on a rack or paper towels. Tempura is best served fresh and hot with a traditional Tentsuyu or dipping sauce, gluten-free soy sauce, or your favorite dipping sauce.

Tentsuyu Dipping Sauce

Heat all the sauce ingredients in a small pan. Set aside to cool. You can serve the sauce in small bowls at the side of everyone's plates.

The thicker the vegetable, the longer it will take to cook. You may want to blanch thicker vegetables (like sweet potato) before frying. Softer vegetables, like mushrooms and eggplant, do not require blanching. Try to cook like-size pieces, to avoid over or under cooking. Cut the vegetables into pieces approximately 1 inch in length, and $1/4$ inch in width. Avoid overcrowding your vegetables, and leave plenty of room to keep them from sticking together. If you use meat, be sure your meat is cooked thoroughly to avoid eating raw or undercooked meat.

When you drop a batter coated veggie in, little pieces of batter will explode off the vegetables, indicating that your batter is hot enough. They should cook for 40 seconds to 1 minute and feel crisp when you move them around with a wooden spoon. You do not need them to be golden brown, so don't wait for that. When you have Crohn's or colitis, it is a good idea to make sure that the vegetables are on the softer side, which will aid in easing digestion.

Examples of suitable vegetables: sweet potatoes, yams, broccoli, carrots, asparagus, mushrooms, zucchini, eggplant, bell peppers, cauliflower. Note that broccoli and cauliflower should be omitted if these vegetables give you gas.

ZOODLES WITH PESTO*

Contributed by Sarah Choueiry
Serves 2
Ingredients:

    1½ pounds of zucchini, roughly 3 big zucchinis

    3 tablespoons of homemade pesto

    Salt and pepper, to taste

    Extra virgin olive oil, to taste

    1 ripe avocado (optional)

Directions:

Peel all the zucchinis and remove the tips. Spiralize the zucchinis and place the zoodles in a large, deep pan on medium heat. Add 3 tablespoons of the pesto and toss until all evenly covered. Cook, stirring around every minute for a total of 10 minutes. You will see liquid release from the zucchini, which is normal.

After around 8 minutes, taste to see if more salt or pepper is needed. Remove the noodles after 10 minutes and retain the liquid the zucchini released. Optionally, drizzle each serving with a little olive oil. Serve with a side of ½ an avocado. It adds an enjoyable creaminess to the pasta, but this is optional.

> I love zoodles. In order to make them, you will need a spiralizer. Not only can you make zucchini noodles with it, but you can also make yam noodles, sweet potato curly fries, and so much more.

HOMEMADE SIMPLE PESTO*

Contributed by Sarah Choueiry

Ingredients:

Half a head of garlic (approximately 10 cloves)

2 cups of tightly packed leaves of basil (from a 4-ounce container)

1 tablespoon lemon juice

1 teaspoon salt

¼ teaspoon pepper

¼ cup extra virgin olive oil

Directions:

Place all of the ingredients except the olive oil in a food processor or blender and blend. Drizzle in olive oil as it blends. Once completely blended, taste it to see if you need more salt or pepper. Makes about 6 tablespoons—perfect for 2 dishes of zoodles with pesto. You can freeze any pesto you do not use in a freezer bag for another night.

I love pesto, but I cannot tolerate the pine nuts or cheese in the traditional recipe. This is great to serve with rice pasta or zoodles, or to bake on top of your favorite fish.

CASHEW SAUCE OVER RICE, BEANS, AND VEGGIES

Ingredients:

Rice

1 cup brown rice

Sauce

¼ cup raw cashews, ground to powder

1½ tablespoons fresh lemon juice

1½ tablespoons nutritional yeast flakes (available at natural food stores)

2 teaspoons sweet white miso or ¼ teaspoon salt or tamari to taste

½ teaspoon onion or garlic powder

¼ cup water (this can be varied, depending on how thick you want your sauce to be)

2 broccoli florets, chopped

½ cabbage, chopped

3 large carrots, chopped

1 bunch kale, chopped

1 can black beans (or ⅔ cup dry beans, cooked, with water until soft)

Grated Parmesan cheese, to taste (optional)

Directions:

Steam or cook the rice. If using a pan, add rice and 2 cups filtered water to a pan. Bring to boil and allow boiling for 1 minute while stirring, then cover, reduce heat to low and simmer for about 10 minutes or until rice has absorbed the water. Stir until the heat is reduced to low.

While the rice is cooking, prepare the cashew sauce by adding all of the ingredients to a food processor or blender. Blend until smooth. Steam vegetables by chopping them large and adding them to a steaming apparatus. Steam until vegetables are soft but still crunchy. Heat beans in a separate pan.

To serve this dish, scoop out rice into a bowl, add steamed vegetables and a serving of beans, then top with cashew sauce. This can be added cold or warm.

THE PERFECT RICE

Contributed by Sarah Choueiry

Serves 2

Ingredients:

    1 cup Calrose rice
    1 cup filtered water (or chicken broth)
    1 teaspoon salt
    1 tablespoon organic, grass-fed butter (or extra virgin olive oil)

Directions:

Soak the rice in a medium-size bowl for one hour. Make sure the water is an inch or two above the rice because the rice will expand. Rinse the rice well under cold water a couple of times and strain. Place the butter in a medium size pot and melt under medium heat.

Once the butter is melted add a cup of filtered water, salt and bring it to a boil. Once boiling, add the strained rice and bring it to a boil again.

After it boils, cover and reduce the heat to a simmer. Let it cook for 10 minutes covered the whole time. After ten minutes, turn the heat off and set the pot of rice aside, covered. Do not open it because you will release the steam. After 5 minutes, you will have the perfect rice.

I was not raised with a rice cooker, but still managed to make great rice every time. This is the way my grandma taught me how to cook rice. Enjoy it with sliced avocados, soup, or just on its own with some gluten-free soy sauce. If you are sensitive to grains, I would avoid this recipe.

TURMERIC LENTILS WITH SPINACH OR CHARD

Ingredients:

- 2 cups red lentils
- 4 cups water
- 1 vegetable bouillon cube, no salt
- 2 tablespoons olive oil
- 1 tablespoon mustard seeds
- 1 onion
- 2 cloves garlic, minced
- 1 tablespoon butter
- 2 teaspoons turmeric
- ½ teaspoon cumin
- 1 teaspoon coriander
- 1 bunch chard, chopped, or 1 large bunch spinach, chopped
- ½ head Napa cabbage (optional)
- 1 pound seasoned chicken sausage, cooked (optional)
- Sea salt, to taste

Directions:

In a saucepan, add lentils, water, and boullion and bring to boil, covered. Reduce heat to medium-low and continue to simmer until all water has been absorbed. This will usually take a little while, so be patient. If all water is absorbed and lentils are not soft, keep adding more water until lentils are soft.

In a separate large saucepan or soup pot, heat olive oil on medium-low heat and add mustard seeds for about 1 minute. Make sure to cover with a lid, because mustard seeds begin to jump once they are hot. Add onion, garlic, and butter and sauté until soft. Add all spices while stirring, and then add chard; add cabbage or chicken sausage, if you are including them. Once vegetables are cooked slightly (but still crunchy) add lentils and cook a little longer until flavors have mingled. Add sea salt to taste and serve over brown rice or quinoa.

COCONUT BROWN RICE

Ingredients:
- 2 cups brown rice
- 4 cups filtered water
- 2–3 tablespoons creamed coconut
- ½ teaspoon pure maple syrup

Directions:
Bring rice and water to a boil in a saucepan. Allow to boil for 2 minutes, reduce heat to low, and then add coconut and maple syrup, cover, and simmer for 15 minutes. Remove from heat and keep covered for another 5 minutes. Serve warm with your favorite vegetable dish.

MUSHROOM RISOTTO WITH CASHEWS AND PARMESAN

Ingredients:
- 1 teaspoon butter
- 2 tablespoons olive oil
- 3 cloves garlic, peeled and crushed with garlic press
- 1½ pounds fresh, wild mushrooms of various kinds (porcini, morels, shiitake, Portobello), cleaned, trimmed, and cut into thin strips
- Pinch of sea salt, to taste
- 1 medium yellow onion, chopped
- 6–7 cups vegetable or chicken broth
- 1½ cups Arborio rice
- ⅓ cup Marsala wine
- ⅔ cup dry white wine
- ⅓ cup Parmesan cheese, grated (optional)
- ½ cup ground cashews
- ½ cup chopped flat leaf parsley

Directions:

Heat the butter and 1 tablespoon of olive oil in a large saucepan over medium heat. Sauté garlic for one minute. Add the mushrooms and sea salt and sauté until the mushrooms release their moisture, get tender, and begin to color around the edges. Heat the remaining tablespoon of olive oil in another saucepan over medium heat and sauté the onion until it is soft and barely golden. At the same time, heat the broth in a soup pan over low heat and keep it warm.

Add the rice to the sautéed onion pan and stir together for a few minutes. Add the Marsala and keep stirring as it reduces, or cooks away. Add the white wine, and after it has reduced, stir in the sautéed mushrooms and about one cup of the hot broth. Adjust the temperature to a low-medium heat so that the broth simmers gently with the rice, and stir slowly as it reduces. When more than half of the broth has reduced, add another cup of the broth while stirring in the same manner. Continue this process until most of the broth is used and the rice is *al dente.* This will take about 20–25 minutes.

When the rice has reached the right texture, stir in the last cup of broth, the Parmesan cheese, and the ground cashews and prepare for serving. Right before serving, add the chopped parsley.

This recipe takes some time to prepare but is definitely worth it! Take the time and you and your guests will be pleasantly impressed.

Staples

HOMEMADE BROWN RICE MILK
Contributed by Sarah Choueiry

Makes two liters
Ingredients:
    ½ cup long grain brown rice
    4 cups water
    Pinch salt

Directions:
Place all of the ingredients in a medium pot, cover and bring to boil. Once it reaches a boil, lower the heat all the way and allow it to simmer for 3 hours. Strain out the rice and discard the water.

Place the rice in a blender and add 2 cups of filtered water for every cup of cooked rice. Blend. Pour the mixture in a cheesecloth-lined, fine strainer placed in a bowl. Grab the corners of the cheesecloth and create a sack, squeezing the remainder of the liquid out. Store the rice milk in a glass container. The brown rice milk will last approximately two weeks in the fridge.

Rice milk is a great alternative to cow's milk. The less you buy boxed and more you create at home, the better. This is my mama's recipe, hope you like it.

HOMEMADE ALMOND MILK*

This is one of my favorites and a go-to drink when I need a dairy alternative.

Ingredients:

1 cup raw almonds

4 cups filtered, alkaline rich water (alternative: basic filtered water is good, too)

1 teaspoon vanilla extract (optional)

4 dates for sweetener or 1 tablespoon honey (optional)

1 pinch salt

Directions:

The night before, soak one cup of almonds in filtered water and let it sit on the counter. Make sure the water covers the almond by at least one inch, as the almonds will expand. Thoroughly rinse out the almonds from the water it had been soaking in, discarding the old water. Place the almonds, water and a pinch of salt into the blender. (Optional: add your honey and/or vanilla extract at this stage.) Blend well on medium power for about 2 to 3 minutes. Line multiple layers of cheesecloth on a fine strainer and place the strainer over a bowl. Pour the almond milk gently into the cheesecloth and slowly lift all sides of the cloth to make a sealed sack.

Squeeze the sack to help release all the extra milk in there. Don't worry about getting your hands dirty. Once everything is squeezed out, refrigerate the almond milk in a closed container. The milk will last for about 3–5 days.

GLUTEN-FREE CORNBREAD

Below is a recipe for a delicious cornbread from my friend Julie Robinson at the Brattleboro Food Co-op.

Ingredients:
- ¼ cup butter, softened
- 2 tablespoons honey
- 2 eggs
- ½ cup dairy-free sour cream or Tofutti®
- ½ cup almond or rice milk
- 1 cup gluten-free flour blend
- ⅔ cup yellow cornmeal
- 2 teaspoons gluten-free baking powder
- ½ teaspoon salt

Directions:
Heat oven to 425°F. Combine butter and honey in a large bowl. Beat at medium speed, scraping the bowl often, until the mixture becomes creamy. Add eggs; mix well. Stir in sour cream and almond milk. Reduce speed to low, adding all remaining ingredients. Beat until mixed.

Pour batter into greased 8-inch square baking pan. Bake for 18-22 minutes, or until golden brown, and a toothpick inserted in the center comes out clean. Serve warm.

BROWN RICE

Ingredients:
- 3 cups brown rice
- Water
- Salt, to taste
- Tamari, wheat-free (for seasoning)
- 1-2 tablespoons sesame seeds

Directions:

Put brown rice and water together in a pot with a lid. Use 1½ cups water for every 1 cup rice. Set the heat to maximum, and bring the rice/water to a boil, uncovered. Then put the lid on the pot, and reduce the heat to low-simmer. If your lid has a steam valve, keep it closed. Let the rice simmer for 20 minutes.

Turn off the heat, and let the rice sit in the covered pot for at least another 10 minutes. If you prefer your rice to be slightly chewy, not mushy, remove the lid after 10 minutes. Be careful when you remove the lid, as a lot of steam may escape when you do so.

I love this recipe and it is my staple for macrobiotic eating. Many people have trouble cooking brown rice and having it turn out decently, since it can be more temperamental than white rice. White rice is a bit easier to digest, but if you cook brown rice this way, it too is easily digested, and is better for you than white rice. If you want to try this recipe for white rice, I like using basmati white rice.

After the rice is cooked, I normally scoop some into a bowl, and mix it with a little tamari and 1–2 tablespoons of sesame seeds. The sesame seeds add a lot of flavor to the rice, but may be hard to digest for some IBDers. I'll also eat it with steamed vegetables, which can be prepared while the rice is cooking. You can store any leftover rice in a plastic container in the refrigerator and it will keep well for several days.

But when I'm not in the mood for cold rice, here's another tasty dish I make from the leftover rice:

In a small pot, add 1 teaspoon of oil (I prefer dark sesame oil because it adds a lot of flavor, but canola oil works well too), and heat it for about 1 minute on medium heat. Add some chopped vegetables (my favorites are onions, green onions, and bell peppers) to the pot, and sauté them in the oil for a few minutes. Once the vegetables are cooked, scoop in some of the leftover brown rice (I like to use 2 parts rice to 1 part vegetables). Mix it well with the vegetables. Reduce the heat slightly, to medium-low, and cook the rice/vegetables for 3–4 minutes until the rice is hot, stirring about once every minute. Pour in a little tamari to taste, and mix it with the rice. Cook for another minute to sear in the flavor. Turn off the heat. Mix in 1–2 tablespoons sesame seeds. Eat and enjoy.

90-MINUTE DRIED BEANS

Ingredients:
    ½ pound dry beans
    ½ tablespoon salt
    Water, to cover

Directions:
Preheat the oven to 250°F. Dump the beans into a large Dutch oven or pot with tight-fitting lid. Pick out any broken pieces. Add the salt. Top with enough water to cover the beans by 1 ½ inches. Bring pot to a boil, then cover the pot and set in the oven. Cook for 75 minutes.

After about 45 minutes in, check the beans. If they look too dry, add some boiling water to the pot. After 75 minutes, the beans should be done—no soaking necessary!

This is my other main staple for the IBD diet! Of all the things I had to give up when I went grain and legume-free, rice and beans were the hardest!

HOMEMADE FARMER'S GOAT CHEESE

Contributed by Sarah Choueiry
Ingredients:
   2 quarts organic goat milk
   ¼ cup apple cider vinegar
   ½ teaspoon salt

Equipment
   Stainless steel pot (big enough to hold the goats' milk)
   Wooden spatula
   Cheesecloth (or a good paper towel over a spaghetti strainer)
   Small round bowl (to pack the cheese into for molding

Directions:
Place the goat milk in a large stainless steel pot and place on medium-high heat. Stir the milk occasionally, making sure to scrape the bottom so nothing sticks or burns. Once it begins to boil, turn off the heat and add the vinegar, stirring a couple times to incorporate it in. You are going to see little curds of cheese forming; let it sit there for 5 minutes.

Place the cheesecloth or paper towel in the spaghetti sifter. Pour the cheese and its liquid into the cheesecloth-lined strainer and with your wooden spoon press down to release all the liquids, draining it. Once drained, place the cheese on a plate and sprinkle salt on top.

Mix the salt into the cheese using a fork and taste. If it needs more salt, add more.

Place the cheese in a small, glass bowl container and pack it in, use the back of a spoon to flatten out the surface. Cover tightly, against the surface of the cheese, with a piece of plastic wrap, and cover with a lid. Place in the fridge. In an hour you can remove the cheese and serve it on a plate with some sun-dried tomatoes or a sprinkle of herbs, whatever you want! As you get more creative, you can place different flavors in the middle of the block of cheese while packing it into your small bowl.

One thing I learned about myself is that I cannot consume most dairy products without my body rebelling. However, I discovered that I can eat goat cheese in moderation without it bothering my system. That being said, I only eat homemade goat cheese; that way, I know how it is being processed and know what I am eating. I recommend avoiding all cheeses if you are currently in a flare or your stomach has been upset lately.

Desserts

⮎

"FRIED" HONEY BANANAS*

Serves 1

Ingredients:

1 organic banana
1 tablespoon organic honey
Coconut oil cooking spray (or 1 teaspoon coconut oil)
¼ teaspoon cinnamon (or more, if desired)

Directions:

Slice the banana into ⅛-inch width. Mix together the honey and ½ tablespoon water in a small bowl and set aside. Place a nonstick frying pan on a medium heat. Spray the pan generously with the coconut oil spray. Allow the oil to heat up, about 1 minute, and then add the bananas. Let the banana cook for about 1–2 minutes, until the bottom is golden brown and then flip.

Once you flip all the pieces of banana over, add the honey/water mixture over the top. Sprinkle the cinnamon on top and enjoy.

> This is Sarah's most popular recipe on The Crohn's Journey Foundation recipe page. It was created during a craving for something sweet in the midst of a Crohn's flare-up. This filled that craving and has always gone down smoothly for me.

COCONUT MACAROONS*

Ingredients:

> 3 cups unsweetened dried coconut flakes
> 1 cup almond meal
> ½ cup raw cacao powder or carob powder (or ½ cup almond meal or coconut flour)
> ½ cup maple syrup
> ¼ cup organic coconut butter
> 1 teaspoon organic vanilla extract
> Pinch of Himalayan salt or sea salt

Directions:

Mix all ingredients together and roll into balls. For a raw dessert, place in dehydrator and dehydrate for 24 hours at a low temperature. To bake, place on greased cookie sheet and bake at 350°F for 8–10 minutes.

ALMOND CAKE WITH BANANA, COCONUT, AND PINEAPPLE PUREE*

Ingredients:

> 2 eggs
> 4 tablespoons honey
> 3 overripe bananas, peeled
> 2¾ cups almond meal
> ½ teaspoon baking powder
> Juice of ½ lemon
> 1 teaspoon vanilla extract
> 2 cups chopped pineapple
> 1 banana
> ½ cup shredded coconut

Directions:

Preheat the oven to 350°F. Generously grease a 9-inch round pie pan. Beat eggs and honey for 10 minutes or until pale and fluffy, then use a fork to mash bananas into this mixture. Add ground almonds and baking powder and stir well. Lastly, stir in the lemon juice and vanilla. Mix until all lumps are dissolved.

Pour into baking pan and bake for 45 minutes or until golden brown on the outside and fork inserted in the middle comes out clean. Remove from the oven and leave in pan on a wire rack until completely cooled.

While cooling, add chopped pineapple, coconut, and banana to blender and blend until smooth. Once cooled, insert knife around all edges to loosen the cake. Invert cake quickly onto a flat plate and ease cake out of the pan. Cover with the pureed mixture and top with fruit to make a flower decoration.

VANILLA CAKE

Ingredients:
   ¾ cup organic butter (or 1 cup coconut oil)
   3½ cups all-purpose gluten-free baking flour
   1¼ cups honey
   4 large hormone-free eggs
   2 teaspoons vanilla extract
   1 tablespoon + 1 teaspoon baking powder
   1 teaspoon baking soda
   1 teaspoon xanthan gum
   1 teaspoon salt
   1½ cups almond milk

Directions:

Preheat oven to 350°F. Lightly oil two 8–9 inch round cake pans and dust with gluten-free flour. Melt butter or coconut oil and beat with honey until it becomes fluffy. Lower the speed and add the eggs, one at a time, while beating. Add vanilla.

In a separate bowl, sift together all the remaining dry ingredients. Add half the dry mixture to the wet mixture and beat on low speed until combined. Then, add the remaining half of the dry ingredients and beat on low speed until smooth.

Divide batter equally between the two prepared pans. Bake in preheated oven for 35–40 minutes or until a fork can be inserted and comes out clean. Cool the cake for 20 minutes in the pans. Insert a knife around the entire edge to loosen the cake from the sides of the pan. Then turn cake over onto wire racks, being very careful when easing the cake out of the pan. Cool completely before frosting. The two cake layers can be layered on top of each other, with or without frosting or filling between the layers.

HONEY VANILLA FROSTING

Ingredients:
    3 egg whites
    ⅔ cup honey
    Pinch of salt
    ½ teaspoon xanthan gum
    1 teaspoon vanilla

Directions:
Put the unbeaten egg whites, honey, and salt into the top of a double boiler over hot water. Beat with an electric beater on medium to high speed, while you bring the water to a boil. As you sprinkle the xanthan gum into the bowl, continue to beat for 7 minutes or until the mixture forms into soft mounds. Remove from heat, add the vanilla slowly and continue beating until frosting is stiff enough to hold its shape. Wait for the frosting to cool before frosting.

CHOCOLATE "ICE CREAM"

Contributed by Sarah Choueiry
Serves 2
Ingredients:

- 2 organic bananas (cut up and placed in the freezer the night before)
- ½ teaspoon pure cacao powder
- 3–4 tablespoons non-dairy milk of your choice

Directions:
Place the bananas, cacao, and non-dairy milk in your blender (you can also use a Magic Bullet blender or a food processor). Blend, pushing down the ingredients with a back of a spoon intermittently. If it is too thick, continue to add your non-dairy milk, 1 tablespoon at a time, until it becomes creamy and thick, similar to a frozen yogurt consistency.

Tip: If you are not a chocolate fan, you can substitute 2–3 frozen strawberries for the cacao powder and create a strawberry/banana ice cream.

> I love sweets, and I am known for having a sweet tooth. This is one of my favorites, especially when it is a hot day, and is great for soothing a craving for a cool dessert. I may not be able to tolerate ice cream, but I can eat this everyday with no issues.

HEALING BLUEBERRY GELATIN

By Jordan Reasoner, Co-Founder of SCD Lifestyle

Ingredients:

1 cup fresh or frozen blueberries (try strawberries too)

3 tablespoons of unflavored grass-fed gelatin

2 tablespoons of fresh-squeezed lemon (or lime) juice

¾ cup SCD yoghurt (or coconut milk kefir)

1 cup hot water

Directions:

Blend berries, yogurt, and lemon (or lime) juice and set aside. Heat water in a pan and slowly melt the gelatin into the water by incorporating a little bit at a time and whisking the water as you temper the gelatin to make sure it melts. Wait for the gelatin-water mixture to cool a bit (so it is not scalding) and add to blended berry mixture and stir well.

Pour your super-food dessert into a container of choice (a 9 × 9 pan works well). Let cool for a couple hours in the fridge until it sets. For a fancy twist you can cut the finished gelatin into cute shapes with a cookie cutter. For extra sweetness, add 1 tablespoon of local raw honey.

Now you can eat your dessert and heal your gut too. No guilt and lots of healing power. Enjoy.

I love eating food that reminds me of being a kid, and Jell-O® is one of those fun foods that takes me right back to my childhood. Gelatin itself is one of the best foods we can eat to heal our gut, which is why we recommend eating bone broth so much.

According to Dr. Siebecker, gelatin is beneficial for the following conditions: "food allergies, dairy indigestion, colic, bean maldigestion, meat maldigestion, grain mal digestion, hypochlorhydria, hyperacidity (gastroesophageal reflux, gastritis, ulcer, hiatal hernia), inflammatory bowel disease (Crohn's disease and ulcerative colitis), irritable bowel syndrome, leaky gut syndrome, malnutrition, weight loss, muscle wasting, cancer, osteoporosis, calcium deficiency and anemia."

Now if you're like me, you can only tolerate so much bone broth, which is why a nice break in the form of blueberry gelatin sounds just right! Thanks to our friend Angela from paleokitchenlab.com for taking the time to share her amazing recipe.

Before we dive in, please note this recipe calls for dairy in the form of 24 hour SCD™ yoghurt. I don't tolerate dairy well, and I've made similar recipes, removing the yoghurt, and it still tastes pretty amazing. So don't let one ingredient stop you from making your own batch.

APPLE CRISP

Chris Ellis, from the Brattleboro Food Co-op, served as the inspiration for this recipe.
Serves 6
Ingredients:
> 6 medium apples, washed and sliced with the skin on, remove seeds
> ¼ cup honey
> ¾ cup almonds (ground up in a food processor until fine)
> 2 cups oats
> ¼ cup honey
> ½ teaspoon cinnamon

Directions:
Preheat an oven to 350°F. Mix the sliced apples and honey. Grind the almonds in a food processor until fine, and then add 2 cups of oats and ¼ cup honey. Continue to process until it looks crumbly.

Take the apple/honey mix and add ½ teaspoon cinnamon and spoon into a greased glass pie pan. Spread the oat/almond/honey mixture over the top and bake for 40 minutes, or until brown. Serve warm or cold.

GLUTEN-FREE APPLE CRISP

Serves 8
Ingredients:
  1 cup oat flour
  1 cup oats
  1 cup brown sugar
  1 teaspoon cinnamon
  ½ cup margarine or butter, cold and diced
  8 cups cored, peeled, sliced apples

Directions:
Preheat oven to 375°F. Mix the first four ingredients, and cut in margarine with a fork to a crumbly consistency. Place apples in greased baking dish, then spread oat mixture on top. Bake for 1 hour, or until bubbly and crispy.

CRABAPPLE WALNUT CAKE

Modified from The Moosewood Cookbook *by Mollie Katzen*
Serves 12
Ingredients:

⅔ cup honey mixed with 2 tablespoons frozen orange juice concentrate (or 1⅓ cups brown sugar)

⅓ cup canola oil

2 eggs

⅓ cup unsweetened applesauce

1 teaspoon vanilla

1 cup almond meal flour

1 cup coconut flour

1 teaspoon baking soda

1 teaspoon cinnamon

½ teaspoon nutmeg

½ teaspoon salt

2 cups apples (Cortland or Macintosh), peeled, cored, and chopped into ¼" pieces

2½–3 cups cranberries

½ cup chopped walnuts (optional)

Directions:
Preheat oven to 350°F. Oil a 9 x 13 inch rectangular cake pan. Blend honey and orange juice concentrate with a mixer at high speed for about 10 minutes, or until it turns white and opaque. Add oil and mix for another minute at high speed. Add eggs, applesauce, and vanilla, and beat well again. If using brown sugar, cream oil and sugar together until well blended and creamy.

Sift flour, baking soda, spices, and salt. Add to the liquid mixture and stir until thoroughly combined. Stir in apples, cranberries, and nuts, and pour into the pan. Bake for 45 minutes, or until toothpick inserted comes out clean.

CONCLUSION

T HE INFORMATION presented in this book is not a definitive guide, nor does it present a cure for IBD. However, one major equation in overall success is patient participation, and you hold the key to your own best life. Having a positive attitude is key!

During the path to health, it is imperative to focus on adequate nutrition, rest, exercise, water, sunshine, and detoxification, while also keeping a positive attitude and setting realistic expectations for yourself. Such ongoing activities and attitudes are the foundations of health. Remember, the goal is to achieve a balance of lifestyle and digestive wellness. It is difficult to actually ask for help, as everyone wants to be successful and function independently. One way to ask for help is to practice with your friends and loved ones. If you are having a bad day and feel like you need to stay by the bathroom, call a friend, or your spouse, and ask them to pick up some ginger tea, rice crackers, and a movie to distract you. You will be surprised at the results!

REACHING OUT

As mentioned above, you will be pleasantly surprised when you reach out to others and ask for help. Take baby steps. For example, if you don't feel comfortable asking a friend for help, call a church group or a "meals-on-wheels" nonprofit agency, and see if you can get some support. Trade with a friend from your support group, if you find one in your area (check the local hospitals for this as many are beginning to offer IBS/IBD support services), and work out a barter. For example, you can say to someone, "I will help you one day a week, or be on call, if you help me."

Talk to your relatives and friends and try to educate them about IBS. Tell them, honestly and without hiding much, how you feel (I know it is hard to talk about diarrhea, but most people will be sympathetic; if not, maybe they should move off your A-list of friends!). It is important that people accept you for who you are, and that you tell them you may need their support for the long haul, and not just for an isolated moment.

FOLLOWING A HEALTHY DIET

Eating well should be a top priority, no matter what your fitness level, age, or health status. You have a responsibility to your body to maintain good health and keep up a stable and beneficial diet. Taking responsibility for this diet is a daily task, and not necessarily an easy one, but staying on track with your eating goals will lead to the overall health you deserve. Always pay attention to your nutrition plan and do everything in your power to stay as close to it as possible.

Keep in mind that there will be days when you will veer off course—this is understandable. Changing your eating habits is a big adjustment; breaking these habits may mean straying from many years' worth of cultural and family habits. Be realistic and honest with yourself; accept that this is a process and that change won't happen overnight. A strong will is a must; no change will occur unless you commit yourself to seeing it happen. By staying optimistic and on-track with your dietary needs, this transitional process will be easier.

Maintaining a healthy diet is not about eating everything you like, and it may require sacrificing some of your less-healthy favorites. Healthy eating is about providing your body with the foods it needs. It is about eating the right amount of calories per day, considering your daily activities. It is about helping yourself in the long run by eating the foods and adapting to the habits that will keep you lively and pain-free.

Eating healthy is also about meal rituals. That means having regular meals at the same times every day. Especially for those suffering from IBS symptoms, scheduled eating times can be extremely beneficial. It is recommended that you eat smaller, more frequent meals throughout the day instead of three or four large meals. You can decide what works for you individually—in many cultures it is customary to walk after a meal, which serves as an aid to digestion! Make sure to always listen to your body, acknowledge your symptoms, and create the appropriate change that will allow your digestive system to function more regularly.

Remember that eating should also be a pleasant experience, and eating well doesn't have to be a daunting task. Fresh fruits and vegetables as well as lean, locally raised, and organic meats (or wild-caught and sustainably harvested fish), when eaten plain or in a delicious recipe, can brighten your day.

FOLLOWING YOUR OWN PATH TO HEALTH

In the last few years, I began to grow some of my own vegetables in my small, raised-bed gardens, and I joined a local Community Support Agriculture (CSA) farm share to augment my vegetable supply and help feed my family. This share was around $350 per year, and included fresh farm eggs—quite reasonable I think compared to buying organic at the supermarket. There is a noticeable growth in farmer's markets and organic gardens and composting centers, like Grow NYC, are seeing unprecedented growth. Clearly, we are on a health path as a nation with Michelle Obama and concerned doctors and health-care practitioners doing their share; however, it is the small and dedicated cadre of patients with Crohn's or colitis, or gluten sensitivity, who are really leading the way. We are demanding and receiving data on diet studies to aid in healing, empowering each other to live life to the fullest, and raising funds through organizations like CCFA.org for research.

I am fortunate to have worked with a naturopathic doctor, who prescribed many herbs, like turmeric, to help me keep inflammation in the small intestine at a low level. The next phase was for me to plan and grow my own herbs at home—there is nothing more satisfying than growing fresh herbs—the fresh smell in the kitchen is enough to please even those olfactory-challenged among us! My vegetable garden is established and expanding, and my herb garden is going in this summer. Even the garlic cloves I planted last fall are coming up in a neat row with no need to replant annually from now on—I will always have fresh garlic. I recently ate fresh asparagus out of my garden, and the tender steamed shoots melted in my mouth.

This new lifestyle is giving me strength and vitality. It is not for everyone—and I always tell people you must proceed with a doctor's advice because Crohn's, ulcerative colitis, and the other autoimmune disease of the large intestine can be serious, even fatal, if not managed correctly. Since Crohn's is persistent, and reputedly cannot be cured, I needed to work with a naturopathic physician, along with my gastroenterologist. This combination of Western medicine and Eastern medicine, along with a more holistic living approach and a strong focus on nutrition has worked well for many people with IBD, and can also be seen as a way to actually prevent diseases like Crohn's and colitis from spreading. Armed with the knowledge given in this book, along with the meal planning guide and a wide assortment of delicious IBD-friendly recipes, you now have everything you need to regain your health and start living life to the fullest!

RESOURCES

ONLINE RESOURCES

A Family Healing Center

www.afamilyhealingcenter.com
Drs. Jason and Jessica Black's full-service Naturopathic clinic.

ABC Homeopathy

www.abchomeopathy.com
Great site to learn about homeopathy that also helps you choose remedies on your own if you want learn more.

American Association of Naturopathic Physicians

www.naturopathic.org
National organization of naturopathic physicians; offers some useful information.

Azure Standard

www.azurestandard.com
This is a site where you can order many natural items at a lesser cost than buying in the store. It does have a minimum order, but you can join others who collectively make orders together in your area.

Bastyr University

www.bastyr.edu
Naturopathic medical school located in Seattle, Washington.

The Center for Food Safety: The True Food Network

www.truefoodnow.org
A resource on current eating trends and how to have healthier diet habits.

Centers for Disease Control and Prevention

www.cdc.gov
This is a site that will help you learn more about diseases, prevalence, acute disease outbreaks, vaccinations, and much more.

The Chopra Center

www.chopra.com
A site for learning how to balance the mind, body, and spirit.

Environmental Protection Agency

www.epa.gov
Great site offering current environmental protection advice relating to foods, environmental concerns, and much more. Their mission is to protect human health and the environment.

Environmental Working Group

www.ewg.org
Wonderful site on environmental toxins and how they are present in our surroundings, and what to do to limit exposure.

Mayo Clinic

www.mayoclinic.com

A site to learn more about various conditions and the current allopathic approach to those conditions.

National College of Natural Medicine

www.ncnm.edu

Naturopathic medical school located in Portland, Oregon.

National Library of Medicine

www.nlm.nih.gov

Oregon Association of Naturopathic Physicians

www.oanp.org

State organization in Oregon for naturopathic physicians.

RESOURCES SPECIFICALLY FOR DIGESTIVE DISEASES

Australia Crohn's & Colitis Association

www.acca.net.au

Caring Bridge

www.caringbridge.org

Free, personalized websites that connect family and friends during a serious illness. Visit www.caringbridge.org/visit/dedecummings to view Dede's personalized site as an example and read more about her personal journey.

The Crohn's & Colitis Foundation of America

www.ccfa.org
A nonprofit, volunteer-driven organization dedicated to finding the cure for Crohn's disease and ulcerative colitis.

Crohn's & Colitis Foundation of Canada

www.ccfc.ca

Crohn's Journey Foundation

www.thecrohnsjourneyfoundation.org
Crohn's Journey Foundation is a nonprofit run for and by individuals with inflammatory bowel disease (IBD). They provide education and support to people with Crohn's disease and ulcerative colitis.

HealingWell.com

www.healingwell.com
Social network and support community. You'll find information, resources, and support, plus full access to the forums and chat rooms.

Irritable Bowel Syndrome Health Center

www.webmd.com/ibs/default.htm

National Digestive Diseases Information Clearinghouse

digestive.niddk.nih.gov/index.htm

Teens with Crohn's Disease

www.ccfa.org/resources/teen-guide.html

NUTRITION RESOURCES

The Paleo Mom
www.thepaleomom.com

Against All Grain
www.againstallgrain.com

Integrative Belly Health
www.integrativebellyhealth.com

AIP (Autoimmune Protocol) Lifestyle: Recipes
aiplifestyle.com/recipe/

Nom Nom Paleo
nomnompaleo.com

Crohn's Journey Foundation: Recips
www.thecrohnsjourneyfoundation.org/recipes/

Specific Carbohydrate Recipes
www.scdrecipe.com

The Specific Carbohydrate Diet Lifestyle
www.SCDLifestyle.com

HELPFUL BOOKS AND DVDS

Andersen Wayne Scott, *Dr A's Habits of Health: The Path to Permanent Weight Control and Optimal Health*, Habits of Health Press, 2009.
Dr. Andersen's book has so much useful information about diet and lifestyle support, plus he has an informative website and e-mails newsletters with useful, weekly tips (for example, get up from your desk and stretch, drink water, etc.).

Black, Jessica K., N.D., *The Anti-Inflammation Diet and Recipe Book: Protect Yourself and Your Family from Heart Disease, Arthritis, Diabetes, Allergies, and More*, Hunter House, 2006.
This book offers excellent recipes that are completely hypoallergenic and anti-inflammatory.

Cumings, Dede and Jessica Black, N.D., *Living With Crohn's & Colitis. A Comprehensive Naturopathic Guide for Complete Digestive Wellness*, Hatherleigh Press 2010.
This book offers excellent recipes that are completely hypoallergenic and anti-inflammatory.

D'Adamo, Peter and Catherine Whitney, *Eat Right for Your Type*, Putnam, 1996.
For individuals who do not know what they are intolerant to, or for those extra sensitive individuals who seem to react to odd foods that are not termed, "inflammatory," other diets might be an option. The *Eat Right for Your Type* Diet was developed by Dr. Peter D'Adamo. He scientifically and elegantly describes how certain foods are better tolerated or more aggravating for an individual depending on that person's blood type. He further discusses particular foods that may be a benefit for some blood types, but can be hindering for others. He describes foods, types of exercises, and even condiments and

seasonings that are more appropriate for individuals based on their blood type.

Eden, Donna, *Energy Medicine: Balancing Your Body's Energies for Optimal Health, Joy, and Vitality*, Tarcher, 2008.
This is such an excellent book, and it can offer many ideas on daily tapping routines to increase the flow of energy in the body and help to make healing possible.

Fallon, Sally, *Nourishing Traditions: The Cookbook that Challenges Politically Correct Nutrition and the Diet Dictocrats*, New Trends Publishing, 1999.
This is a cookbook and an excellent resource if you want to learn how to begin making more homemade fermented foods.

Gates, Donna and Linda Schatz, *The Body Ecology Diet: Recovering Your Health and Rebuilding Your Immunity*, Body Ecology, 2006.
This book discusses increasing gastrointestinal resistance and overall health by the use of probiotics.

Gershon, Michael D., *Second Brain: The Scientific Basis of Gut Instinct and a Groundbreaking New Understanding: of Nervous Disorders of the Stomach and Intestine*, Harper-Collins, 1998.
A book that explores the enteric nervous system, otherwise known as the brain of the gut, sometimes with humor.

Gottschall, Elaine Gloria, *Breaking the Vicious Cycle: Intestinal Health Through Diet*, Kirkton Press, 1994.
Investigates the link between food and such intestinal disorders as Crohn's disease, ulcerative colitis, diverticulitis, celiac disease, cystic fibrosis, and chronic diarrhea.

Kamm, Laura Alden, *Intuitive Wellness: Using Your Body's Inner Wisdom to Heal*, Atria Books/Beyond Words, 2006.

Laura Alden Kamm endured her own personal health journey and came out on the "other side," as she relates in her remarkable memoir.

Kinderlehrer, Jane, *Confessions of a Sneaky Organic Cook or, How to Make Your Family Healthy When They're Not Looking!*, New American Library, 1972.
This is an older book but has so many good ideas in it. Usually you can find one used online for a very inexpensive price.

Lair, Cythia, *Feeding the Whole Family: Cooking with Whole Foods*, Sasquatch Books, 2008.
This is a fun book that gives many ideas on quick meals for the family.

Remen, Rachel Naomi, M.D., *Kitchen Table Wisdom: Stories that Heal*, Riverhead Trade Books, 1997.
Remen is one of a growing number of physicians exploring the spiritual dimension of the healing arts.

Santorelli, Saki, *Heal Thy Self: Lessons on Mindfulness in Medicine*, Three Rivers Press, 2000.
Santorelli, director of the Stress Reduction Clinic at the University of Massachusetts Medical Center, does a wonderful job with this book, and it is one of Dede's favorites for aiding her recovery. Santorelli guides the reader through the process of learning to listen to our bodies, and bringing mindfulness into our lives. Most of the patients in the Stress Reduction Clinic have never meditated, or been involved in groups or alternative therapies, so his work, and that of the clinic's founder, Jon Kabat-Zinn, is highly regarded and a model of success.

Scala, James, *The New Eating Right for a Bad Gut: The Complete Nutritional Guide to Ileitis, Colitis, Crohn's Disease, and Inflammatory Bowel Disease*, Plume, 2000.
Dr. Scala's book was one of Dede's first purchases at her local used bookstore after diagnosis. His advice and step-by-step dietary guide-

lines are enhanced by his clear and concise education in eating a healthy diet. A great complement to a learning library.

Straus, Martha B., *No-Talk Therapy for Children and Adolescents*, W.W. Norton, 1999.
Straus opens for readers a huge grab bag of gimmicks, gadgets, and games from which to draw resources appropriate to every no-talk occasion. This book will be useful for parents or caregivers of younger IBD patients who struggle with a lack of language with which to express their emotions.

Weil, Andrew, *8 Weeks to Optimum Health: A Proven Program for taking Full Advantage of Your Body's Natural Healing Power*, Ballantine Books, 2007.
Dr. Weil is one of our "health gurus" and, again, a great book and website resource.

Yee, Rodney. *A.M. and P.M. Yoga.* DVD. Director: Steve Adams. Rating: NR (not rated.)
Yee, Rodney. *Moving Toward Balance: 8 weeks of Yoga with Rodney Yee*, Rodale Books, 2004.
Rodney is Dede's "yoga guru" and arguably one of the most important influences on her improved overall health. Together with his wife, Colleen, he teaches yoga on Long Island at "Yoga Shanti" studio. Rodney continues to be supportive of the mind/body connection in health and well-being, offering encouragement to the authors, as well as to his many students. His website: www.yeeyoga.com.

GARDENING

GARDENING IS NOT FOR EVERYONE, but you never will know unless you try it. My advice is to start small. I hope this section inspires you to look at your own backyard, patio, rooftop, or sunny windowbox, and consider a garden. Since I have eliminated grains and dairy from my diet, I eat mostly fruits, veggies, nuts, and animal protein (eggs, chicken, and occasional fish). Summer is the best time to do this diet: organic fruits and veggies are readily available, and meat that is local, antibiotic-free, and grass-fed is plentiful. I plan on putting up and preserving a lot of extra produce at the end of the growing season, so I can continue summer's bounty from my freezer (and canning room) during the cold Vermont winter. Growing your own food is another way to reduce stress and get physically fit—gardening is good for upper body strength! Here I will outline some of the basics for getting started, and remember, if you live in a city, you can do a community garden, or even start by growing herbs and tomato plants in containers.

Pick a Site

- Look for a site that meets your garden's purpose and goals. When choosing the potential garden site, keep in mind several considerations, including:
- Light: At least 6 hours of direct sun daily.
- Drainage: Little to no standing water after heavy rains.
- Slope: As level as possible.
- Exposure: Protected from high winds; Avoid low-lying frost pockets.
- Surrounding vegetation: Few trees; Look out for problematic plants (i.e. poison ivy, stinging nettles).
- Soil: Test the soil for heavy metals and other contaminants. Most regional agricultural extension universities provide services for soil testing
- Water: Ideally a close water source should be available.
- Safety: If digging, make sure not to dig on a utility line; Call "811" Before You Dig.
- Accessibility: Location and layout of site should be suitable for the gardener and for bringing materials onto the site.
- Size: Space large enough for the number of potential gardeners, garden infrastructure, a diversity of garden activities, and room for growth.

How to Build a Raised Bed

The instructions provided below are just one way to build a raised garden bed. Many other designs have proven successful. If 4 in. x 4 in. timbers are hard to come by, try using 2 in. x 8 in. boards or other sizes that may lower your cost. If you are using thinner boards you can use long screws rather than timber ties, which can be less expensive.

Depending on your garden needs, you may also want to consider a shorter or higher raised bed design. In terms of wood used, hemlock is often used in New England for its longevity, decent price, and availability. Cedar and wood/plastic composite are also options, buy can be prohibitively expensive. Most importantly, do not use pressure treated wood if you are using the beds for food gardens.

Supplies:

- Circular saw and accompanying safety equipment
- Square (tool)
- Level
- Measuring tape
- Pencil
- Shovels
- Hammer
- Scissors
- Wheelbarrow or buckets

Twelve 8-foot 4" x 4" timbers are needed to assemble a 4-layer, 4 ft. x 8 ft. raised bed. The lumber will be stacked and each layer will overlap the layer below it at the corners. Here are the four different measurements to prepare:

- First, trim all timbers to the maximum possible common length, as they may not all be exactly 8 feet. Set aside four boards. These will be used for the sides of layers 1 and 3.
- Measure the width of a timber (as it may not be exactly 4 inches). Double this width and subtract from the length of the timbers cut in step 1. This will be the length to cut the four timbers used for the sides of layers 2 and 4.
- The end pieces of layers 2 and 4 are made by cutting two timbers in half.
- Subtract the doubled timber width from the length of the end pieces of layers 2 and 4. This will be the length to cut the two boards used for the ends of layers 1 and 3.

*Note: A simpler option is to cut all the timbers to the maximum possible common length, then cut four timbers in half for the ends and follow the stacking process as outlined below. The bed will end up slightly larger than 4 ft. x 8 ft.

The first layer is the most important as all other layers are built on it. The raised bed box will be sturdiest if the first layer is dug into the ground. Use a square and level to ensure that the first layer is as square as possible.

If the area under the raised bed is grass, the sod can be stripped and composted. If the soil underneath the raised bed is determined by a soil test to have contaminants and/or heavy metals, a layer of landscape fabric can be put under the bed as a semi-permeable barrier that excess water in the bed can seep through. When constructing the frame, each layer is nailed to the layer below it using large 6-inch galvanized timber ties, spaced every 16 inches. You can also use 4-inch galvanized screws and a drill to nail the boards to a corner post.

The final step is to fill the raised beds with a topsoil/compost mix. Starting a garden this way takes a lot of time and a bit of an expense initially, but it should last for years and produce a relatively weed-free garden bed.

COMPOST AS MULCH

The forest floor is a natural composting system in which leaves are mulch on the soil surface, and then gradually decompose, recycling nutrients and conditioning the soil. Likewise, yard debris such as leaves, grass clippings, or shredded branches can be used as mulch in the landscape and allowed to compost on the soil surface. Over time, the mulch will compost in place.

Finished or unfinished compost can be applied as a mulch 3 to 4 inches thick on the soil surface. Do not incorporate into the soil. Keep compost mulch 2 to 3 inches away from plant stems. Nutrients will filter into soil, without robbing nitrogen from the root zone. Compost offers similar benefits to regular mulch: soil moisture retention, insulation of soil from extreme temperatures, soil breakdown to provide nutrients, and organic matter for soil structure.

One disadvantage to using compost as mulch is that it will not act as a barrier to weed growth, but in fact will promote weed growth if not covered with a standard mulch material. Compost or mulch should be reapplied yearly to replenish the decomposing layer.

COMPOST AS POTTING MIX

Compost can be used as an excellent potting soil for your container nursery. Compost offers good water retention qualities and some basic nutrients. However, gardeners should use only fully decomposed (called "finished") compost as a potting mix.

Container grown plants need a potting soil that retains moisture, but is well drained. Most gardening enthusiasts blend compost with coarse sand, perlite, vermiculite, etc. to make optimal planting media.

If your compost still has large chunks in it, but is otherwise finished, you may want to screen the compost through a ½-inch screen to remove un-decomposed material that could rob nitrogen from the plant roots. Leaving some coarse or bulky material in the mix will help maintain a well-drained planting media.

RECIPE INDEX

ABOUT THE CONTRIBUTORS

SARAH CHOUEIRY'S STORY

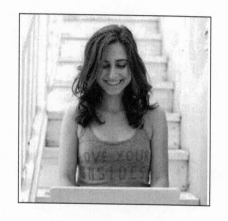

Each time before I begin my daily meditation, I ask myself three questions:

1. Who am I?
2. What is my purpose?
3. What do I want?

Who am I?

My answer is, simply, "I am Sarah Choueiry—a daughter, wife, and friend to many. I'm an advocate, a lover, and a woman on a journey." I have to be honest and admit that it wasn't easy finding the clarity necessary to answer that question. It took me a long time to realize that being a "sick" person—a "Crohnie"—is a part of who I am but it does not define me. What I represent is love, hope, and truth—not illness and the anger and frustration that initially came with it. I am someone who hopes to inspire others to explore alternative ways to find healing; and in this book, I share my philosophy with diet, which is only one part in my journey to health.

What is my purpose?

I have dedicated my life to achieving and spreading good health through love, compassion and education. I love to cook, go to yoga, bond with good friends, spend time with my family and continue to educate myself on things that can better my health.

I am a speech and language pathologist, and as of two years ago, a proud founder of the non-profit, The Crohn's Journey Foundation. I was diagnosed with an inflammatory bowel disease (IBD) called Crohn's disease at the age of twelve. Because I was so young, I didn't understand the struggles I would face for years to come—and I had no idea how important my journey would become to myself and others.

I created The Crohn's Journey Foundation to not only share my journey, but to educate patients and caregivers who are struggling with the devastating effects of Crohn's disease and ulcerative colitis. The foundation helps those with IBD find healing peace through a healthy balance of Eastern and Western medicine.

I continue to strive to grow and share my journey with others, hoping to inspire, motivate and bring light to many diagnosed with Crohn's disease and ulcerative colitis.

What do I want?

This is the simplest answer and pretty self-explanatory. I want happiness, health, success, and love. You can never go wrong if you have all four in your life!

Where does cooking fit in?

Now that you know a little about my background, let's get back to cooking! My philosophy with cooking is quite similar to my philosophy in life:

- Keep things simple with minimal stress
- Have fun!
- Surround yourself with high-quality people
- Avoid all things that cause inflammation (e.g. stress, foods, people, jobs, etc.)

This is not easy to do at times, and is truly a journey—one I was blessed to have been given, because without Crohn's, I do not think the sweet would be as sweet and the gratitude I have developed for life as abundant.

DEDE CUMMINGS' STORY

Who am I? Crohn's patient, mother, hiker, author. I have Crohn's disease, which is a disease of the small intestine and is not curable, according to the Western medicine world. I surprised my doctor, and have had seven years of clinical remission after a bowel resection in 2006. These last seven years have been filled with hope and health, though at times it can be easy to fall into despair when the doctors tell you that your disease has gone from nonexistent to "severe."

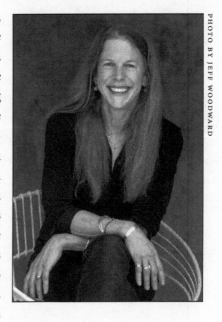

PHOTO BY JEFF WOODWARD

Rather than saying "Woe is me," and spending time feeling sad and useless (I did a lot of that, believe me), I decided to take action, and try to live by the words of the Dalai Lama:

"Scientists say that a healthy mind is a major factor for a healthy body. If you're serious about your health, think and take most concern for your peace of mind. That's very, very important."

In following those wise words, I am now on my way to health—my primary goal has been to stay focused and take care of my body: better food, sleep, stress relief, education, awareness, team building, satisfying work, making money enough to live on, giving back to my community and the world, and working for peace, justice, and environmental sustainability.

Our IBD community is growing, which is a sad fact. According to the CDC, Crohn's disease and ulcerative colitis are on the rise exponentially accross the board in the United States and in the developed world. Slowing down our lives, taking time to learn about our bodies, our minds and our spirits, is key to overall health and well-being, not sure for ourselves, but for our planet.

NOTES FROM YOUR DOCTOR/GI CLINIC

NOTES FROM YOUR DOCTOR/GI CLINIC

NOTES FROM YOUR DOCTOR/NATUROPATH

NOTES FROM YOUR DOCTOR/NATUROPATH

NOTES FROM YOUR DOCTOR/NATUROPATH

NOTES/SHOPPING LIST/SUPPLEMENTS

NOTES/SHOPPING LIST/SUPPLEMENTS